SLEEP WITHOUT BACK PAIN

Pascal Mannekens

SLEEP WITHOUT BACK PAIN

Choose the right bed
and maximize your
comfort and sleep

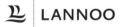 LANNOO

Contents

Ten test questions

Before you begin reading this book, I would like to ask you to first of all reflect on your own mattress and sleep quality. In the following ten questions, mark each answer that best fits your sleeping situation.

1. When I'm lying in bed:
   - ☐ I can easily find a comfortable sleeping position and I fall asleep quickly;
   - ☐ I lie tossing and turning for a while.

2. When I lie stretched out in bed:
   - ☐ my head and feet remain within the mattress dimensions.
   - ☐ my feet touch the end of the bed.

3. When I turn over:
   - ☐ my partner doesn't feel me turning over and stays asleep.
   - ☐ my partner feels me turning over or rolls towards me.

4. When I lie on my side:
   - ☐ the mattress, bed base and pillow support my entire body;
   - ☐ my bed feels hard or it feels like I'm lying in a dip.

5. When I lie on my back:
   - ☐ lying stretched out feels comfortable and relaxed;
   - ☐ it feels like my legs are raised or it feels like I'm lying in a dip.

6. When I wake up in the morning:
   - ☐ I have no neck and/or back pain;
   - ☐ I have at least one of the following: numb hands or arms, shoulder pain, mild headaches or a sensitive neck.

7. When I get up:
   - ☐ my legs and back feel relaxed;
   - ☐ I have somewhat stiff and aching legs and an aching feeling in my lower back.

8. 8. When I get up:
   - ☐ I feel fresh, well rested and I can get up without difficulty;
   - ☐ I am still tired, not well rested and getting up is an effort.

9. When I look at my mattress:
   - ☐ it looks fresh and clean;
   - ☐ it appears grimy, spotted and lumpy (with depressions).

10. I have been using my current mattress:
    - ☐ for less than ten years;
    - ☐ for more than ten years.

Were you able to mark the top answer nine or ten times?
Congratulations on the quality of your sleep and your mattress!

Did you choose the top answer eight times or less?
Then it's probably time for you to get more information about a sleep system that better suits your body and your sleeping habits.

Back pain: not a disease but a symptom

Back complaints and sleep disorders are evolving worldwide into one of the major social problems: 60 to 80 percent of the Western population will be faced, in the course of their life, with a moment of non-specific lower back pain, with a peak between the ages of 35 and 55. In 85 percent of the cases, no clear cause for the presence of the pain can be found. In America, the cost of treating patients with chronic back pain exceeds $90 billion a year!

Approximately 50 to 70 percent of patients with chronic lower back pain have sleep disorders. If you suffer from a sleep disorder but do not have back pain, it is even assumed that those sleeping problems may be a risk factor for the subsequent development of back pain. For the time being, it is still unclear to what extent sleep disorders are the cause of lower back pain or vice versa, or to what extent they are both the result of other causes.

But it cannot be denied that a problem exists. In the United Kingdom alone, 120 million working days are lost every year as a consequence of back pain. In Japan, back pain, shoulder aching and arthrosis are amongst the most frequently reported complaints among the population.

Meanwhile, the back is now our second most common location for pain. Back pain is not a disease but a symptom.

Based on my scientific background as a physical therapist, researcher and experienced expert in guiding thousands of patients in the quest to maximize their sleep comfort, I felt the need to convey my knowledge about the right bed for your back.

I want to explain to everyone why a good bed is so important for your back and for your night's sleep. It is disconcerting to see how little most people know about their sleep system – the combination of mattress, bed base and pillow – especially when you consider that we spend a third of our lives in our bed, and that it has such a big influence on our quality of life.

Therefore, in *Sleep without back pain*, I want to dispel the many misunderstandings and prejudices about beds. This is also in line with one of the main guidelines of the European working group on the prevention of back problems, COST Action B13, namely that back patients should be properly informed about fundamental care for the back, which we will call back hygiene.

Good back and sleep hygiene with adequate treatment of pain is one of the pillars for the treatment of back and neck patients. This implies that therapists must apply maximum effort to every kind of prevention. You cannot resolve poor sleep with medication (although medication may temporarily be part of the treatment). Discuss this with your general practitioner.

An important part of treating back patients with sleep disorders is related to education about sleep (what you need to know about sleep), sleep hygiene (what you should not do or conversely what you should do), back hygiene and relaxation-related therapies. The focus of the treatment must therefore simultaneously be on back pain as well as on sleep disorders.

Sleep without back pain aspires to be a guide that accompanies you in your quest for the best bed for your back. But even if you are not immediately planning to buy a new bed system, you can probably considerably increase your sleep comfort by means of the many tips that I give in this book.

After reading this book you will have a better understanding of the interplay between your body and your bed.

Happy reading and sleep well!

CHAPTER 1

How our back is put together

Chances are that at some time or another you have been troubled by back pain. Over 80 percent of all people will experience this at some point in their life. So you have only one chance in five that you will escape back pain.

Usually, it involves lower back complaints caused by incorrect positions and movements – in other words, by incorrect strain on the spinal column. Because those are mechanical factors, doctors often speak of mechanical lower back pain. This you may already experience at a young age, especially if your occupation involves a lot of sitting or standing.

To gain an understanding of how lower back pain arises, we first need to take a closer look at the structure of the back and the spinal column.

THE SPINAL COLUMN

The spinal column is the central support axis of our skeleton. It supports the body and protects our organs.

Much is demanded of the spinal column: it needs to be sturdy, or we would not be able to stand upright without problems. At the same time, it must also remain flexible, otherwise we would not be able to move our trunk. How the spinal column manages to meet those two opposing requirements will be revealed below.

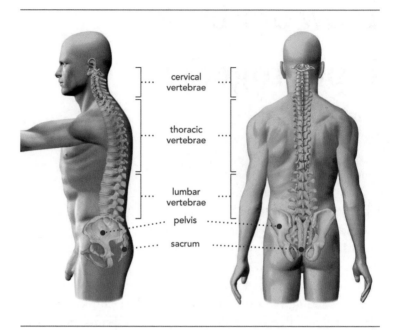

Figures 1 and 2   The spinal column in lateral and posterior view.

We have 24 distinct vertebrae, which are divided into three groups. The seven **cervical vertebrae** are relatively small. They support the head, which weighs about seven kilograms. Below are the twelve **thoracic vertebrae**, to which the twelve ribs are attached. The rib cage protects organs such as the heart, the lungs and the liver. Further down are the five **lumbar vertebrae**. They are large and sturdy because they must bear a substantial part of the body weight – 80 percent when we are standing upright. The lowest lumbar vertebra is connected to the sacrum. The sacrum consists of five fused vertebrae and, together with the hip bones, forms the pelvis. The pelvis is the base of the spinal column and the upper body. It also connects the spinal column to the legs, and protects the abdominal organs, the bladder and the sexual organs.

From side view, the spinal column has a natural S-shape. This enables the spine to carry the weight of the upper body and helps to absorb shocks. A normal spinal column has four curves (Figure 1): the cervical curve forwards at the neck, the thoracic curve backwards at chest level, the lumbar curve forwards at the lower back and the sacral curve backwards.

THE VERTEBRAE

Now that we know the structure of the spinal column, we can elaborate on the elements of which it is composed: the vertebrae.

In Figures 3 and 4, you can see that a vertebra consists of three parts: on the front side is the vertebral body located, in the middle, the spinal canal and on the back side, the vertebral arch, which is equipped with joints and protrusions.

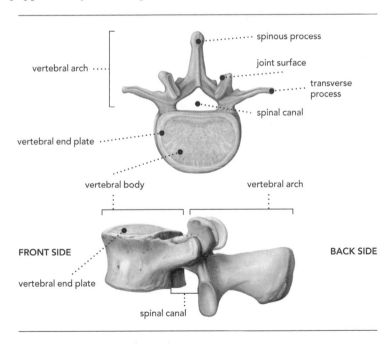

Figures 3 and 4   Structure of a vertebra.

The **vertebral body** is the largest bony part of the vertebra. It has the shape of a disc and is somewhat flattened at the rear. At the top and bottom, it is covered with a thin layer of cartilage – we call those layers the vertebral end plates.

Seen from above, each vertebra has an opening between the vertebral body and the vertebral arch. All together, these openings form the **spinal canal**: a tunnel through which the spinal cord passes.

On the rear side of the **vertebral arch**, we notice several protrusions. Some of those, together with the corresponding protrusions of the adjacent vertebra, form the four facet joints. They are held together by a joint capsule and ligaments, and make bending and stretching of the vertebrae possible. Bending, we have a convex back, stretching, a concave one. The facet joints direct these movements as well. Rotating movements are possible within limitations. The facet joints carry 15 to 20 percent of the weight that is supported by the spinal column.

You feel the large protrusions on the back of the vertebrae as bumps on your back. We call those the spinous process. To the left and to the right are the transverse processes located. Spinous and transverse processes are the levers with which the vertebrae are moved: they constitute anchor points for ligaments and muscles.

THE INTER-VERTEBRAL DISC

Between two vertebral bodies there is a flat disc that serves as a shock absorber and as a stabiliser. This disc absorbs the majority of the forces loading our backs as we walk, run, jump or perform other everyday activities. The inter-vertebral disc is composed of cartilage, connective tissue and for 80 to 85 percent of water. It does not lie loose between the vertebrae, but is firmly attached.

The inter-vertebral disc has two components: the annulus, the outer peel, and a nucleus.

The **annulus** is made up of ten to twelve concentric rings of tough connective fiber, which are firmly attached to the vertebral bodies and the ligament structures. The function of those rings of connective tissue is mainly to absorb tensile forces. They are also capable of processing the twisting forces as we turn our trunk and they dispense 25 percent of the compressive load on the inter-vertebral discs.

The jelly **core** (Figure 5) of the inter-vertebral disc absorbs the remaining 75 percent of the compressive load. At birth, the core consists of 85 to 90 percent of water. Later on, this amount decreases to about 70 percent. Thanks to this flexible core, the inter-vertebral disc can change shape and perfectly follow the movements of the vertebrae.

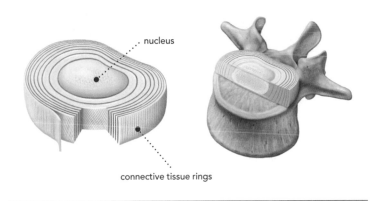

nucleus

connective tissue rings

Figure 5   Detailed cross-section of an inter-vertebral disc.

Every minute of our lives, our inter-vertebral discs are under strain. The Swedish back researcher Alf Nachemson measured the pressure on the third lumbar inter-vertebral disc in various standing and lying positions. The results are shown in Figure 6.

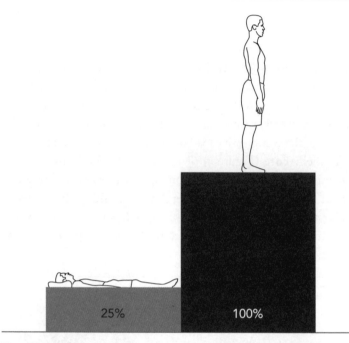

Figure 6 Relative decrease in the pressure on the inter-vertebral disc in a supine position compared to the pressure when standing upright. The pressure is expressed in percentages of the body weight (100 percent = body weight).

When we are standing upright, the pressure on the inter-vertebral disc is found to be approximately equal to the body weight. Let's just call it 100 percent. As soon as we lie down, the pressure does drop, but it never goes away completely – in the supine position, we will still find it to be 25 percent.

At the level of the lumbar vertebrae, the spinal column is curved forwards. The pressure is therefore partially directed forwards onto the connective tissue rings that are located on the anterior side. The nucleus, which is shifted somewhat forward, and the rear connective tissue rings are less heavily loaded. In order to compensate for the uneven distribution of pressure, the inter-vertebral disc is thicker at the front side and significantly thinner on the back side (see Figure 7).

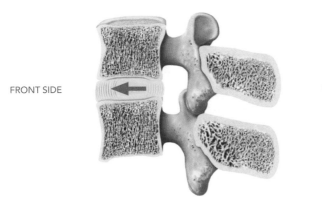

FRONT SIDE

BACK SIDE

Figure 7   The inter-vertebral disc is significantly thicker on the front side.

The inter-vertebral disc consists mainly of cartilage and connective tissue, and has no blood supply. Having no blood supply has the advantage that it can absorb forces without bleeding, but it makes the supply of nutrients slow, because those now have to seep in from the surrounding ligaments. This takes place primarily by diffusion through the end plates of the adjacent vertebrae. That is also why inter-vertebral discs heal slowly. Moving a lot at daytime and adopting various positions will keep your inter-vertebral discs in good condition and will improve the supply of important nutrients.

THE LIGAMENTS

The facet joints in our spinal column are supported by tough, rigid fibrous bands: the ligaments (see Figure 8). These ligaments keep the joints firmly together and limit great movements. In addition, very strong ligaments also pass over the entire length of the spinal column, on both the front and back sides. Their main function is to stabilise the spinal column and protect it against harmful extreme movements.

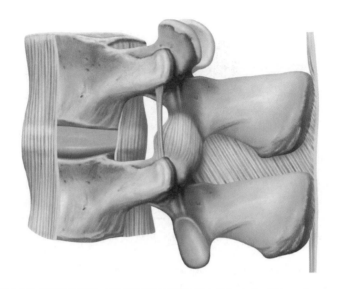

Figure 8   Ligaments of the spinal column.

Ligaments heal more difficult if they become damaged: substances which are needed to heal must be supplied via the blood, and ligaments have only a limited blood supply. What's more, the healed ligament will never again function as well as before the damage: the fibers cling together and form scar tissue, which gives rise to reduced elasticity.

THE MUSCLES

All vertebrae together form a flexible column – which is so flexible that it cannot keep itself upright: therefore it needs help from the muscles. One can compare it somewhat to the tall mast of a sailing ship: it can only remain upright with the help of cables that exert forces in different directions (Figure 9).

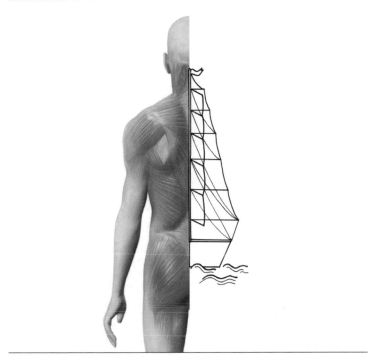

Figure 9　Muscles function like the cables of a sailing ship, where we can compare the mast to the spinal column.

To begin with, we have **short back muscles**, which run from one vertebra to another. On the one hand, they make very subtle movements possible, and on the other hand, they also limit movements. They serve mainly to maintain **positions**. On top of those little muscles run **long back muscles**, which span a large part of the spinal column. In thin people those are clearly visible. They serve mainly for the **movements** of the trunk. Together with the abdominal muscles, the back muscles form a sort of natural corset. The better the muscles control and coordinate movements, the stronger and more capable of bearing loads our back becomes. Buttock and leg muscles are also important for the back and must be in good condition. They play an important supporting role in all sorts of postural and movement patterns.

THE NERVOUS SYSTEM

Our nervous system is traditionally divided into a central and a peripheral part.

The **central nervous system** consists of the brain and the spinal cord. It is surrounded and protected by bony structures: the skull and the spinal column.

The **peripheral nervous system** connects the brain and the spinal cord with the rest of the body – it contains all the nerves running outside our skull and spinal column.

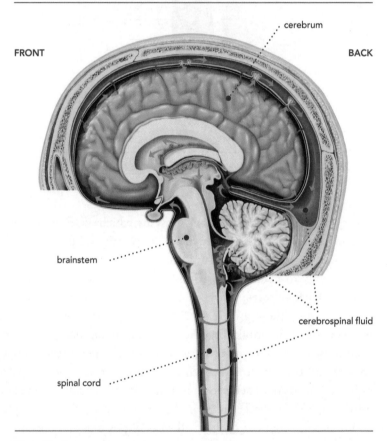

Figure 10   The central nervous system.

CHAPTER 1

The central nervous system

Let's first take a somewhat closer look at the central nervous system. As you can see in Figure 10, the brain is connected to the spinal cord via the brainstem – the lower portion of the brainstem merges without any clear boundary into the spinal cord.

In adult humans, the spinal cord is 16 to 18 inches long. It hangs like a kind of cord below the brain and is surrounded by two soft connective tissue membranes and one hard membrane, the dura mater, also called the dura (see Figure 11). Those spinal cord membranes are the continuation of our meninges. Fluid between those membranes dampens shocks and acts as an extra buffer. The dura is attached at the top to the skull and at the bottom to the sacrum. It is extremely sensitive to pressure and pain.

The peripheral nervous system

Twelve cranial nerves, mainly serving the head, depart from the brainstem. They process sensory information and facilitate movements such as those of the eyes and facial muscles.

Originating from the spinal cord are four nerve bundles between each vertebra, two on both sides. They join together at the level of the inter-vertebral foramen, to form a spinal nerve. Every human being has 31 pairs of them. The dura has shoots – also known as dural sleeves – that cover the spinal nerve until somewhere beyond the inter-vertebral foramen (Figure 11).

Messages go back and forth via the spinal nerves and spinal cord between our brain and the rest of our body. The brain can, for instance, give our leg muscles the command to contract and, conversely, it can receive information about temperature or pain from our hands.

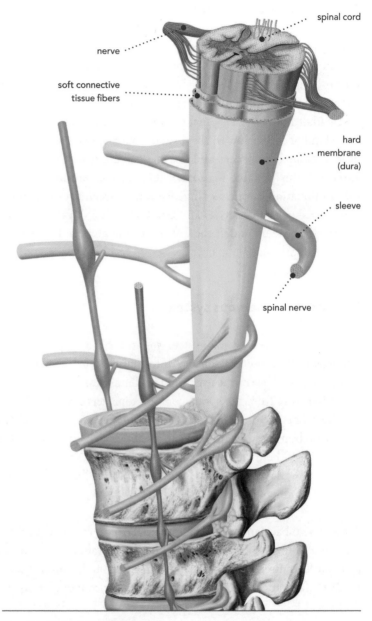

spinal cord

nerve

soft connective
tissue fibers

hard
membrane
(dura)

sleeve

spinal nerve

Figure 11   The peripheral nervous system.

THE FUNCTIONAL UNIT

Now, been taught about all the parts of the spinal column, it is time to put this information together and see how all the parts work together. We can best do this by further examination of the functional unit.

A functional unit consists of two adjacent vertebrae. All of the parts – bones, joints, inter-vertebral disc, ligaments, muscles and nerves – work together to make the spinal column a strong, rigid structure that can still easily change shape, providing the best possible protection for the vulnerable spinal cord.

We can divide the functional unit into three compartments, each with its own task (Figure 12).

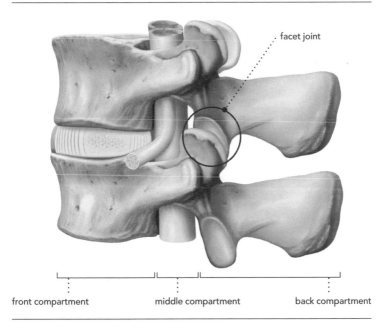

facet joint

front compartment   middle compartment   back compartment

Figure 12 The functional unit.

The *anterior compartment*, on the front side, consists of the vertebral body and the inter-vertebral disc. It carries the largest part of the body weight and serves mainly to absorb shocks.

The *middle compartment* is the spinal canal: it protects the spinal cord and the roots of the spinal nerves.

The *posterior compartment*, on the rear side, consists of the vertebral arch and the facet joints on that arch. Its main function is to direct and facilitate movements.

What causes back pain?

The spinal column is a very clever unit of mechanics, a complex edifice of very diverse elements which fit together beautifully. We never give it a moment's thought, until one day we feel pain in the back. In this chapter, we will find out where the pain comes from, and what causes it.

Lower back pain is very common. Most people are likely to experience this at some time in the course of their lifetime. Not illogical: the lower back – at the level of our lumbar vertebrae – bears most of our body weight and is therefore the most heavily loaded.

Not only is the pain annoying, but you also experience discomfort when performing everyday activities. Your doctor will probably talk about normal non-specific lower back pain. Non-specific means that no specific physical cause can be discerned – once you've read through this chapter, you'll understand what that means. The term 'normal' indicates that it is about local injuries that, unlike tumors and so, are not life-threatening. Lower back pain is not a disease but a symptom, possibly of quite a few mechanisms.

WHERE DOES IT HURT?

In a mechanical system, the points at the pivot of the movement are almost always the most vulnerable. In comparison with a door, for instance, the hinges are the first to suffer damage: every time a door is opened or closed the hinges wear out a little, and even when the door is not moving, the hinges still have to carry the weight of the door.

Our back is no different. When we expose the spinal column to uneven, prolonged or heavy loads, can this lead to damage of the inter-vertebral disc, the ligaments, the facet joints and the muscles between and around the vertebrae. Scientists believe that the inter-vertebral disc plays a direct role in 80 percent of all of mechanical back pain. Facet joints, muscles and ligaments are responsible for the remaining 20 percent.

Bending, stretching and turning

The main causes of lower back pain are one-sided long-term strains on the spinal column. They can arise from poor positions when we sleep, or when, for instance, we are sitting on an office chair that is too low. Incorrect movements are also a major cause: for instance, lifting a crate of beer by bending from the waist in-stead of bending the knees. It is better to distribute pressure across all the joints in our body in a back-friendly way. For tips or advice on this you can consult a physical therapist or an ergonomic occu-pational therapist.

To better understand what can go wrong, we need to look more closely at what positions the spinal column can assume, and what injuries that may lead to.

» Bending

Our spinal column can curve forwards. When we sleep in a ham-mock on our back or when we bend forwards while sitting, we assume such a **curved position**. We carry out a **flexion** or bending movement when we stoop. Both times, while in this position and while perform-ing this movement, our back is convex (Figure 13).

This creates a flexion load or a bending load: the space between two vertebrae becomes wider on the back side and more narrow at the front. The facet joints at the back of the vertebra open up, which creates a high tensile strain in the rear fibers of the connective tissue rings – these are in fact connected to the vertebral plates that are moving away from each other. At the same time, the connective tissue rings on the front side are compressed, which in turn pushes the nucleus backwards and imparts compressive stress to the connective tissue rings on the back side (Figure 13). With repeated movements and as the years go by, all those forces together will cause small fissures in the connective tissue rings.

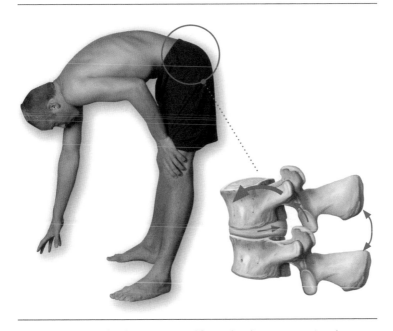

Figure 13 With both bending positions and flexion (bending movements), we have a convex back.

» Stretching

The opposite position is called stretching. An example of such a **position** is lying face down in a hammock; an example of a **stretching movement or extension** is painting the ceiling (Figure 14). In both cases, the back is concave.

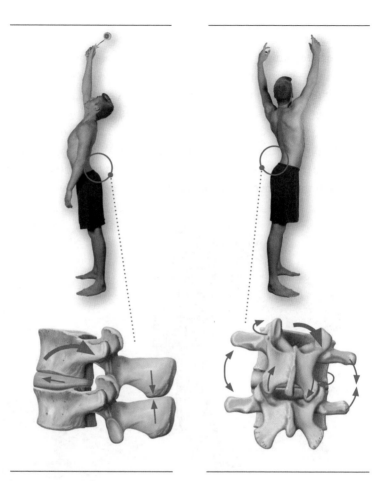

Figure 14 When stretching we have a concave back.

Figure 15 Turning (rotation) can also lead to injuries.

Extension or stretch loading arises: the facet joints of the vertebrae are closing, the front of the connective tissue rings is put under tension, the rear side is compressed, and the nucleus moves forwards (Figure 14). Over the years, this can lead to injuries. Usually, this causes no intervertebral disc problems, because the connective tissue rings in the front are very sturdy. The increased pressure on the facet joints causes pain. This is known as facet pain or joint capsule pain. In addition, pinched nerves at the level of the spinal nerve root canal can also cause a lot of trouble.

» Turning

Finally, the vertebrae can rotate around their axes by turning or torsion. Lying on your stomach horizontally on a flat bed with your
shoulders horizontal and your pelvis vertical is an example of such
a **position**. A good example of **movement** is the most classic of all
gymnastic exercises: with raised arms, turning your trunk first to the
left and then to the right (Figure 15).

Again, excessive load or wear and tear over the years can lead to
injuries. Rotation overload can best be compared with wringing out
a cloth: the fluid is squized out, so to speak, from the inter-vertebral
discs and the ligaments come under increased pressure (Figure 15).

DISORDERS OF THE INTER-VERTEBRAL DISC

Now that we have come to know the positions of the spinal column a
little, it is time to find out how the parts of our vertebrae are affected
by these. We will start with the inter-vertebral disc, because presuma-
bly this is the cause of about 80 percent of all lower back pain.

We generally divide disorders of the inter-vertebral discs into two
categories: primary and secondary discogenic disease. Discogenic
means originating from the inter-vertebral disc.

Primary discogenic disease (PDD)

In a primary discogenic disease or PDD, sprains or fissures arise in
the inter-vertebral disc. That can happen all of a sudden, for instance
while performing an uncontrolled movement, but often it is a result
of increased tissue fatigue – wear and tear.

This usually involves damage to the connective tissue rings, both
on the back and on the lateral side. The rear fibers of the connective tissue rings are thinner and consequently more vulnerable to
damage. They are also subjected to more stress in combined bending

and rotational movements. Sitting and standing up from a sitting position is usually more painful than walking and standing. Patients with a PDD are usually younger than 45.

Such wear may go unnoticed for a long time when the fissures start at the core and then gradually spread to the outer connective tissue rings. Only the outer circles of the connective tissue rings are in fact equipped with sensory nerves and blood vessels. So only if the injury has reached those outer circles will you feel pain (Figure 16). When the connective tissue rings are torn from the outside, pain will be felt at once.

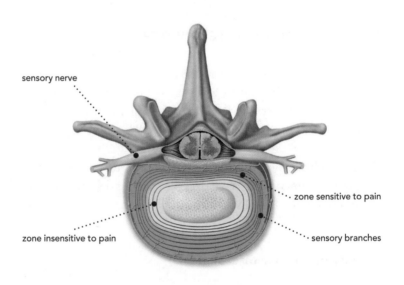

Figure 16   Zones of the inter-vertebral disc sensitive to pain (red) versus insensitive to pain.

When the inter-vertebral discs are fissured, the bending stiffness decreases, the middle zone increases, and other structures such as ligaments may become overloaded so that they also fissure or strain. When those inter-vertebral disc fissures are limited to the pain-insensitive inner connective tissue rings, it is quite possible that you will first feel the pain in the ligaments, and only much later in the inter-vertebral disc. The tissue damage will cause an immediate inflammatory response. This is the first stage of the recovery process. After that, growth factors ensure that new connective tissue forms and that the damage is repaired. However, that newly formed tissue is less strong, which immediately brings us to secondary discogenic disease.

Secondary discogenic disease (SDD)

A secondary discogenic disease (SDD) is caused by scars left by PDDs. As we have just seen, these scars form weak spots and can easily fissure again. If this happens more than once in a short time, it can disrupt the function of the core, and eventually of the entire inter-vertebral disc.

SDD manifests primarily in older people. Due to the thinning of the inter-vertebral disc, the facet joints will come to be more heavily loaded, which will also cause them to wear out faster. In the long term, this leads to exostosis, arthrosis of the facet joints and possible narrowing of the spinal canal and the inter-vertebral disc spaces. SDD is especially painful in the case of extension strain when the back is concave.

THE MOST COMMON COMPLAINTS

There are many names for back pain, and in common language, they often tend to be used mixed. We will now point out the most commonly used terms.

» Lumbago
If you feel a sudden back pain, for instance, after a wrong movement, we call that lumbago. This too is sometimes called back pain or backache. The pain 'shoots' into the back, usually on one side. Such an attack of acute back pain generally subsides spontaneously after one

or two weeks. Lumbago is usually caused by overloading of the spinal column, when sitting or lying incorrectly. The name refers to any sudden lower back pain, and says nothing about the physical cause: that may be any of the structures of the motion segment. The pain always remains local: there is no radiation.

Primary discogenic disease (PDD)

» Disc protrusion

When you repeatedly put tension on your back incorrectly, the fibers of the connective tissue rings will tear over time. This renders the rings less sturdy and, eventually, material from the nucleus or core will seep through the fibers. If the natural recovery process is no longer able to contain the damage, the gelatinous core is at this point only being restrained. Doctors call that a disc protrusion – the medical term for the bulging of the inter-vertebral disc (see Figure 17).

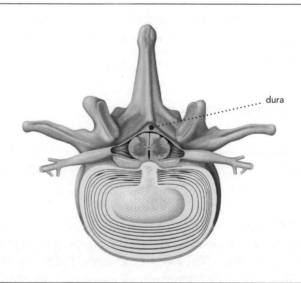
dura

Figure 17 Central disc protrusion with pressure on the hard spinal cord membrane (dura).

We feel pain when the protrusion presses against a pain-sensitive structure. A central disc protrusion, for instance, can irritate the connection between the connective tissue rings and the posterior longitudinal ligament, which runs vertically over the entire back side of our spinal column.

It may even press against the dura mater, a hard membrane that envelops our spinal cord (Figure 17). The pain is now not limited to the back anymore, but radiates over the buttocks and thighs, and possibly to the lower legs.

If the inter-vertebral disc protrudes more laterally, it can put pressure on the nerve root where it emerges from the vertebra (Figure 18). The symptoms are now localized more at the left or right side of the back, and can radiate to the buttock area or even to the upper leg. Patients complain of a strange, numb feeling with a tingling feeling in the legs. With more severe pressure on the nerve root, loss of strength in the leg may even occur. Doctors describe these symptoms as the 'radicular syndrome'.

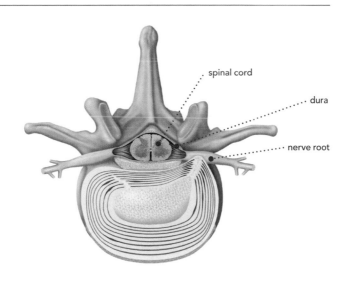

Figure 18   If the inter-vertebral disc protrudes more laterally, we call it dorsolateral protrusion.

» Hernia or disc prolapse

A hernia is caused by a poorly healing disc protrusion: the bulging material breaks through the outermost fibers of the connective tissue rings and forms a bulge. Incidentally, it is not the nucleus that bulges, as has been often wrongly assumed and as is still too often suggested: research has proven that it often concerns newly formed connective tissue.

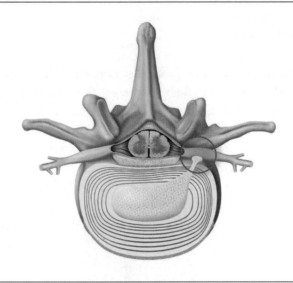

Figure 19 Inflammation of a poorly healing disc protrusion, better known as a hernia.

If the bulge is large, it may press directly on the nerve root, which causes a strong inflammatory response (see Figure 19).

The patient feels a sharp and clearly localised pain, sometimes with radiation to the legs. Doctors call shooting pain from the back with radiation to the leg 'radicular pain'.

The pain is worsened by coughing, sneezing and straining, and is more pronounced while sitting than while standing and usually disappears when the patient lies down in the correct position. The pressure on the nerve root can be so heavy that reduced power (e.g. in the feet), sensory disturbances (tingling), and diminished reflexes occur.

The symptoms of a 'radicular syndrome' are thus often combined with those of 'radicular pain'.

Sciatica is a term that refers to the pressure that a hernia exerts on the nerve roots. These, together with the peripheral nerve, will form the sciatic (also rarely referred to as the ischial) nerve (see Figure 20). Nervus ischiadicus is the medical term for the large lower limb nerve. In a severe inflammatory reaction, the pain will appear in the back, the buttock and sometimes even in the whole leg following the course of the sciatic nerve.

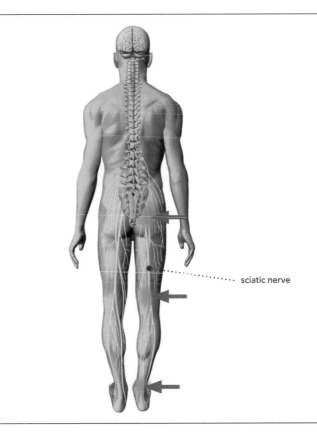

sciatic nerve

Figure 20   Course of the large lower limb nerve (sciatic nerve) with indication of the key pain zones.

The transitional phase between PDD and SDD: from disc degeneration to facet pain

The nucleus of the inter-vertebral disc consists for the most part of water. As we age, that moisture content decreases and the disc diminishes. In a newborn baby, the moisture content is 90 percent. In people over 70, the moisture content is often only 70 percent. Until we are about 30 years old, we hardly notice any consequence of that dehydration process. After this age, the dehydration process can play a role in the development of lower back pain.

The connective tissue rings also wear out over the years: the fibers become less elastic, which makes it even more difficult for the nucleus to retain moisture. Movement is important for the maintenance of the nutritional mechanism of the inter-vertebral disc. Rest makes you rusty!

With prolonged uneven tension on the inter-vertebral disc, the core will be displaced. If, for instance, you lie on your back in a hammock, the nucleus will slide backwards. Water and dissolved materials will move from the most heavily loaded side to the least heavily loaded side. We believe that this slows down the rehydration of the inter-vertebral disc, which eventually can lead to even greater wear.

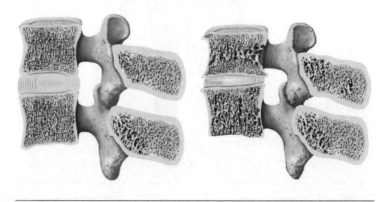

Figure 21 A healthy inter-vertebral disc (left) versus a worn out inter-vertebral disc (right).

The final result is that the inter-vertebral disc collapses – such narrowing of the inter-vertebral disc can be seen on x-ray. We call this process disc degeneration or wear to the inter-vertebral disc. The inter-vertebral discs that are the most loaded will shrink the most rapidly (see Figure 21).

Due to the narrowing of the inter-vertebral disc, the vertebrae come lie closer to one another and come under much greater pressure (Figure 22). The joint protrusions sag on top of each other. As a result, the space through which the nerve roots run may narrow. This will obviously lead to pain. The facet joints themselves will become irritated and the joint capsule will swell and can also put pressure on a nerve.

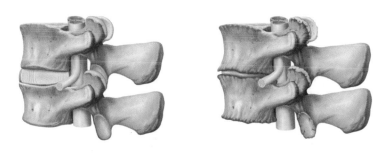

Figure 22   A healthy spinal column segment (left) versus a spinal column segment subjected to wear (right).

Disc degeneration also will lead to heavier load on the facet joints. The joint capsules and ligaments are richly supplied with nerves, which can lead to pain. That pain is called facet joint pain or facet joint capsule pain. Facet degeneration may also occur without any degeneration of the inter-vertebral disc.

The fact that over the years the vertebrae come to lie closer to each other and the flexion rigidity of the inter-vertebral discs decreases also affects the ligaments. These come to be less tightly stretched and will slacken. That means that the joints will loosen up – they are given more space to move, thereby increasing the possibility of shifting the joint surfaces relative to each other. This can cause blocking of the joint.

Secondary discogenic disease (SDD)

» Arthrosis

Over time, the facet joint itself will wear out (Figure 23). The medical term for this is arthrosis: cartilage is lost, the bone hardens beneath the cartilage, and the joint capsule could become inflamed. In arthrosis, the disc wear is also clearly visible. Small uncontrolled growth of the bone, exostosis could also develop at the edge of the joint.

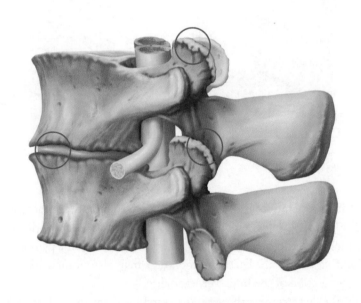

Figure 23   Wear of the facet joint with exostosis and narrowing of the inter-vertebral disc.

» Degenerative spinal stenosis

Spinal stenosis is the medical term for narrowing of the spinal canal. The classical patient is a man who is middle-aged or older, who has had back pain for years and more recently feels radiation in one or both legs.

The initial pain is caused by a narrowing of the inter-vertebral disc, as we have seen above. Exostosis and shifts of the vertebrae may then exert pressure on the dura mater in the central spinal canal (Figure 24) or in the inter-vertebral spaces through which the spinal nerves run. This causes lower back pain with radiation into the legs. The clinical picture resembles a hernia, but its treatment is different. A herniated disc is temporary, but once patients are suffering from degenerative spinal stenosis, they cannot get rid of it anymore.

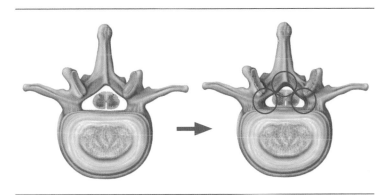

Figure 24   Normal spinal canal (left) and central canal stenosis (right) with exostosis and arthrosis of the facet joints.

PAY ATTENTION: CREEP!

How does soft tissue like ligaments and inter-vertebral discs actually wear out? This has everything to do with collagen, an elastic protein that forms an important part of human connective tissue and plays a major role in the transmission of force.

In our spinal column, collagen-containing connective tissue is present in inter-vertebral discs, ligaments and joint capsules. When the connective tissue is loaded and put under tension, it stretches. If this tension persists for a long time – for instance, if you sleep on your side in a hammock – then the connective tissue will gradually elongate. You can compare this with a tightened clothes line: over time, it will also lose its elasticity, with the result that it elongates and starts to hang loose.

This lengthening of the connective tissue is called *creep*. The connective tissue 'creeps' ever further. But unlike carrier straps, connective tissue can recover if it gets sufficient rest. The more slack it shows, the more time it will need to recover.

During this recovery period, the connective tissue is longer and less elastic, and this has an influence on its functioning. Ligaments help, among other things, to control movements from the facet joints. Functional impairment will affect those movements and will cause stiffness, pain symptoms and locking of joints.

Nice to know: the brain will give the command to increase muscle tension around the injury to prevent additional damage – which is a natural protection mechanism. For instance, the neck stiffness that one feels after a whiplash is a form of *bracing*. An acute back stiffness after an injury of the inter-vertebral disc is also an example of muscle tension, protecting you from more damage.

Inter-vertebral discs are also provided with collagen connective tissue, and that too can exhibit slack. We all have, at some time, experienced some stiffness getting out of a car after a long drive: this is due to the prolonged static tension on ligaments, muscles tissue and inter-vertebral discs.

For collagen connective tissue to be under tension during the day is normal – that's what it is for – but at night it must be able to rest and recover. That is why a good sleep system is so important. Anyone who sleeps in a bed that is too hard or too soft not only prohibits the connective tissue to get the rest it needs, but puts even more strain on it during the hours it ought to be recovering!

If the connective tissue is strained year in and year out and does not get time to recover, the symptoms can become chronic. Blockages in the cervical spine because of neck-straining positions are an example of that.

NEURAL STRUCTURES

Earlier we talked about pain that occurs in soft tissue. Now we want to talk about symptoms related to neural structures.

Surrounding the spinal cord is a strong, pain-sensitive membrane, the dura mater, or dura for short. The dura together with the ligaments is fixed to the vertebral bodies. The dura also encloses the nerve roots that emerge from the spinal cord. This is important, because the nerve roots get their nutrients from the dura (Figure 25).

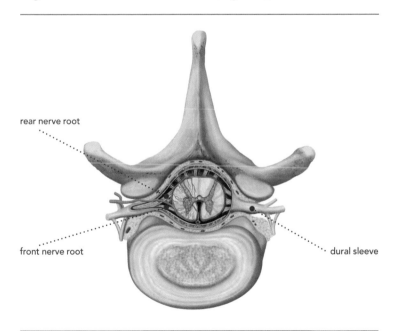

rear nerve root

front nerve root

dural sleeve

Figure 25   The nerve roots obtain their nutrients from the dura and the dural sleeve.

When flexing the spinal column, for instance when lying on the back in a hammock, the spinal cord and the dura are stretched, causing a slight decrease in the cross-sectional area – comparable with a rubber band becoming thinner when you stretch it. As a result, the tension in the spinal cord and the dura increases over the entire length of the spinal column. Only when a nerve is inflamed and the blood supply and agility of the nerve are greatly reduced, can it result in pain.

Upon overstretching the spinal column – for instance, lying on the stomach in a hammock – the spinal cord and dura are pushed into each other: their cross-sectional area expands, and creases arise. This is not painful in itself. However, pressure on the facet joints may happen and nerve roots leaving the spinal cord may become pinched at the level of the nerve root openings. If, for instance, you are lying on your right side in a hammock, the nerve root openings on the left side of the vertebrae will become smaller. This can cause pain.

NON-SPECIFIC LOWER BACK PAIN

Meanwhile, you probably figured out why doctors talk about non-specific lower back pain. Injuries originate mainly due to wear and repetitive or repeated incorrect positions and movements. Often they start at the inter-vertebral disc, but all the other components of the motion segment will also be affected by it. Therefore the pain can not be traced back to one specific, well-defined point. The parts of our vertebrae are far too interconnected for that.

CHAPTER 3

The relationship between sleep and back complaints

We all know how important a good night's sleep is in order to be able to start a new day feeling fit and energetic. This also applies to our spinal column: all day long it carries the weight of the body, so at night it must be able to recover from that heavy task. It is vital that the spinall column is then loaded as little as possible.

It seems logical that back pain leads to sleep disorders. Some scientists argue that the reverse is also true. Impossible to state clearly what the correlation is, but we know for sure that there is a close link between sleeping problems and back pain. In this chapter we will talk about that interdependence. We will begin with a not so obvious question.

WHAT ACTUALLY IS SLEEP?

Adult human beings typically have one major period of sleep in 24 hours – that is the natural rhythm of our body. 'Sleep' has to do with how living beings have by evolution adapted to recuperate efficiently, within the system of day and night. It is also known that night rest has a beneficial effect on our memory, on our central nervous system and on the processing of knowledge. It is estimated that more than 30 percent of adults in the Western world suffer from sleep disorder.

Sleep quality can be measured with a hypnogram or sleep curve. To do this, four body signals are recorded simultaneously: eye movement, muscle tension, heart activity and brain activity. When we bring all this information together, we get a nice picture of the stages of sleep that we go through every night (Figure 26).

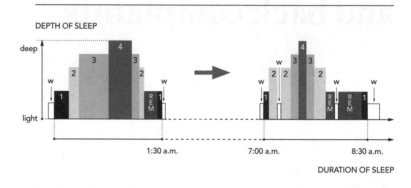

Figure 26   Sleep curve with the relationship between the first sleep cycle (with mainly deep sleep, stages 3 and 4) and the last sleep cycle (with mainly REM or dream sleep and more wakefulness recordings, W).

REM AND NON-REM

There are two types of sleep that alternate with a certain regularity: REM sleep and Non-REM sleep. REM stands for *rapid eye movement*, the rapid eye movements that occasionally occur in that stage. During REM sleep, we almost always have vivid dreams, so this stage is also sometimes referred to as dream sleep. The brain is very active: it shows a similar, non-identical pattern as during daytime. For instance, it seems as if the brain is processing lots of visual and auditory information, and it also conveys movement instructions to the body. Fortunately, those signals are suppressed,

48

otherwise we would jump out of bed and perform the actions that we are dreaming of. Researchers assume that REM sleep is the fundamental, biological stage of sleep. Indeed, without REM sleep, we would die.

By Non-REM sleep, we mean the periods of sleep that are characterised, among other things, by decreased brain activity and little or no occurrence of eye movements (see Figure 27).

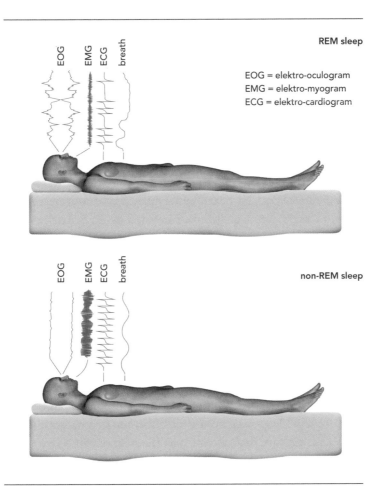

Figure 27   Differences in physiological responses between REM and non-REM sleep.

FIVE STAGES

Normal sleep is made up of an average of four to six cycles, each lasting 90 to 100 minutes. Each cycle is again subdivided into five stages (see Figure 26).

The first stage is falling asleep. We call the period of time that elapses from getting into bed until stage one the sleep onset latency. Normally this takes five to 15 minutes, and it is a reasonable predictor of sleep quality: the shorter the sleep onset latency, the better the sleep. In stage one – the scientific name is N_1 – the eyes make slow, rolling movements and muscle tension reduces (the force exerted by the muscles at rest on the attachment points). There may be short dreamlike experiences and brain activity slows down. At stage one, most people do not really feel that they have already fallen asleep.

Stage two, also referred to as the pre-sleep, lasts ten to twenty-five minutes. Muscle tone decreases further and the slow rolling eye movements cease. The heart and respiratory rates decrease as does blood pressure. You can still be awakened easily. Scientists call this stage N_2.

Approximately 30 minutes after falling asleep, we come at **stage three**, and another 15 minutes later at **stage four**. There are some quantitative differences between those two stages, but they are usually treated as one stage – researchers name it N_3. Muscle tone decreases even further, just like the heart and respiratory rate and blood pressure. If you wish to wake up someone in stage three or four, you need very strong stimuli, hence the term 'deep sleep' or 'core sleep'. During deep sleep, growth hormones are produced, and our body repairs itself. Deep sleep occurs mostly in the first half of the night's rest. It makes sure that we can start the next day fit – if you do not feel fully rested during the following day, that's probably because you haven't had enough deep sleep.

After stage four, we go back through stage three to stage two again. During stages three and two, especially just before REM sleep, strong muscle tensions are often measured, because we are changing our lying position more frequently. The sleep seems to become more superficial and the brain begins to show stage-one-like activity.

Instead of waking up, about one hour and 45 minutes after falling asleep, we go into REM sleep. Breathing becomes uneven, as does the heart rate, which slows down or may even speed up by 40 percent.

In the course of the night, there is a regular alternation between Non-REM sleep and REM sleep. Every 90 minutes we go through a REM stage. The first one lasts five to ten minutes, subsequent ones get increasingly longer. In the stage before waking up, we are already at 45 to 60 minutes. REM sleep and stage two predominate in the second part of the night. At that point we have shorter periods when we are awake. Researchers record that on the sleep curve as stage W (see Figure 26).

In a normal young adult, sleep on average consists of 5 to 10 percent N1, 50 percent N2, 20 to 25 percent stage N3, and 20 percent REM sleep (see diagram below).

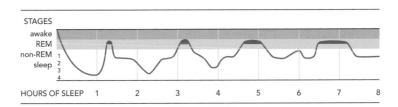

After each cycle we thus arrive at **stage W**, in which we briefly wake up – without being aware of it. Stage W usually introduces the start of a new cycle, though we also record stage W during the stages, for instance, when we change position during those stages. On average, we have 7 to 10 W recordings per night. If there is no noise, if the room temperature is not too high or too low, if the bed is comfortable, the pillow still offers support, in other words if there are no disturbing elements, we will fall asleep immediately.

The transition from REM sleep to in-between stage W is an important time for people with back problems: if they wake up briefly after a REM stage, it is possible that because of the pain, they will not be able to fall back asleep.

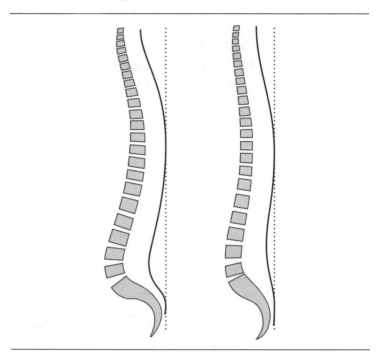

Figure 28   Spinal column when upright (left) and spinal column with smoothed curves when lying down (right).

THE INFLUENCE OF SLEEP AND LYING DOWN ON LOWER BACK PAIN

During sleep, the heavy burden on the inter-vertebral discs ceases. This gives them the opportunity to absorb moisture, so that they regain elasticity. Also the pressure on the facet joints is reduced, so that the cartilage can nourish itself. In the morning, we are approximately three quarters of an inch taller than in the evening. This is partly because the curves in our spinal column are somewhat more flattened and because the inter-vertebral discs have absorbed moisture and thus have become thicker (see Figure 28).

If the spinal column is properly supported during sleep, soft tissue such as ligaments, nerves and blood vessels also relax. The muscles relax, the heart needs to perform less in order to pump blood around the body and because of the decreased brain activity, we feel less pain. Both, tissue damage and pain related to this, generally decrease at night.

INSOMNIA

Fifty to 70 percent of patients with chronic lower back pain exhibit sleep disorders. This usually refers to insomnia or sleeplessness: patients have more difficulty falling asleep, wake up often and in the morning they feel not fully rested. We often assume that this is due to back problems – they are unable to find a comfortable position for falling asleep and when they wake up during the night, they cannot fall back asleep because of the pain. A Finnish scientist suggested that we ought to look at the matter from the other way around: he determined that sleep disorders are a risk factor for the development of lower back pain. And these arguments make sense: anyone who sleeps poorly will have a lower pain threshold and thus feel pain more readily. In addition, we know that people with low self-esteem and who sleep poorly are more likely to develop back pain later in life.

In any case, educating patients is now an essential part of treating sleep disorders and back pain. In this book we will also give tips about sleep and back hygiene. Especially the interaction between the body and the bed will be extensively discussed.

THE IMPORTANCE OF A GOOD SLEEP SYSTEM

We would like to point out that a good sleep system plays a major role in maintaining a healthy back and reducing complaints of pain. Many studies point in that direction: for instance, results from a Dutch survey and a private study clearly show that a relationship exists between the bed and neck and back aches, shoulder pain and pain in the morning. We also know that chronic back pain patients with sleep disturbances sleep better on a comfortable mattress. Ninety-five percent of American back surgeons further confirm that the quality of the sleep system has a significant beneficial effect on the well-being of their patients. A person who sleeps on an unsuitable system also has a greater likelihood of recurring neck and back problems.

Actually, it makes perfect sense: all sorts of things happen to your body when you fall asleep: your muscles relax, you are no longer aware of your surroundings, your body temperature drops... That means that your sleep system is very important: it must facilitate a good, undisturbed night's rest, and support and protect your body night after night.

In the following chapters, we take a closer look at how to put an optimal sleep system together.

The basics of a good bed

Conformity, hardness, thermal insulation and humidity regulation: those four properties of the bed are essential for a good night's sleep. In this chapter we will deal with these one by one. We will conclude with a list of things you definitely should pay attention to if you are planning to purchase a new bed.

CONFORMITY

Conformity indicates how well your sleep system adapts to your body shape, taking into account the distribution of your weight over your body (Figure 29).

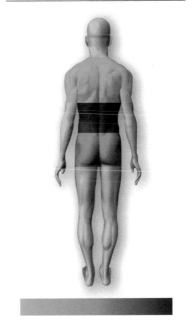

Figure 29 Three important zones with variable weight, whereby the shoulder zone of the body (light green) is less heavy compared to the middle zone of the body (dark green).

LIGHT   HEAVY

It is a very important criterion, because the position of the spinal column will be determined to a large extent by the degree of conformity. As we have seen in Chapter 1, the spinal column forms a straight line if we view it from the front or the rear. Viewed from the side, it has an S-shape, with four curves.

Very important: if you sleep on your side, the spinal column should keep to the horizontal line as much as possible; when lying on your back, the natural S-shape should be maintained (Figure 30). This would ideally also be the case while lying on your stomach, but even with a very good sleep system, this is not so obvious. Fortunately, most people do not often lie on their stomach.

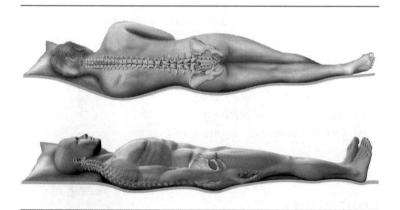

Figure 30 Sleep system with good conformity and correct support of the spinal column in supine and lateral positions.

A good sleep system will therefore have to give way just enough: not too much, nor too little. When you lie on the back, it should give way somewhat at the level of the shoulders and hips, but on the contrary, should support the neck, waist and legs. When you lie on the side, it is primarily the shoulders and the hips that should be well accommodated.

The conformity of the sleep system depends to a large extent on the elasticity and flexibility of your mattress – we can define elasticity as the speed at which the material yields when it is pressed in or assumes the original shape when it springs back. If, for instance, you switch from lying on your left side to lying on your right side, the parts of your mattress that are no longer bearing weight should immediately bounce back. The parts that do carry your weight now should give way immediately. If that happens too slowly, your body will not be sufficiently supported and it wil be difficult to find a stable position. The degree of elasticity also helps to determine the hardness.

A bed which conforms too little will do violence to the normal position of the spinal column. This leads in the long term to deflections of the spinal column, which can cause severe back pain (Figure 31). Conformity therefore not only has a major influence on the comfort of lying down, but it is also important for the health of the back.

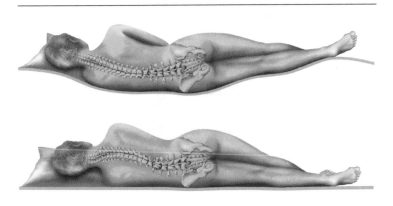

Figure 31 Two examples of poorly conforming beds with poor support of the spinal column. The top sleep system is too soft; the bottom sleep system is too hard.

When buying a sleep system, try it out in all positions. In any event, check whether your spinal column forms a straight line when lying on your side. The position of the shoulders and hips is important in that respect: they protrude somewhat compared to the rest of your body, and they should also sink into the bed to the same extent.

HARDNESS

Hardness indicates how deeply we sink into the mattress. With the same load, a soft mattress will thus be more deeply indented than a hard mattress.

Heavier people will benefit from a hard mattress: they sink too deeply into a soft mattress. The body must then exert too much force in order to change position, which leads to a great loss of energy during the night.

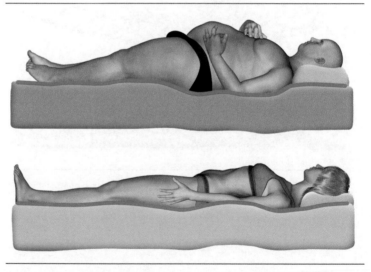

Figure 32 Heavy people should always sleep on a harder mattress rather than a lightweight one. It would be best for the man at the top to opt for a hard mattress, the woman below to opt for a soft mattress.

Lightweight people sleep best on a somewhat softer mattress (see Figure 32).

Hardness was formerly related to the *body mass index* (BMI) of the sleeper – the ratio between the weight and the (square of) the height. Nowadays, we also take into account the distribution of weight over the body. There ought to be harder mattress segments underneath the heavier body parts.

✗ Mud and bouncing balls

For those who have some difficulty distinguishing the concepts of conformity and hardness: the degree of conformity indicates how well the sleep system adapts to your body shape; hardness indicates how deeply the system is indented per unit of weight. A hard mattress, for instance, can offer high conformity for an obese sleeper, but none whatsoever for a lightweight individual.

And for anyone who doesn't immediately grasp the difference between hardness/softness and elasticity: mud is soft but not elastic – mud does not recoil. A bouncy ball is hard and elastic, but a table top is hard and not elastic.

Hardness is certainly also a question of personal preferences. We often choose a mattress based on what we are used to, or because friends or family have recommended a certain type to us. But the fact that they sleep well on a particular type of mattress does not mean that the same will apply to you. Habituation can lead to a preference that doesn't entirely suit you – only you don't realise that because you are unaware of the other possibilities!

HEAT INSULATION

People are heat generators: we constantly produce heat. During sleep, we emit a small portion of it by way of respiration and the majority of it through the skin. If the insulation values of our sleep system and bed linen are too low, we will lose more heat than we produce. We then cool off, which encourages muscle stiffness and sleep disorders. If the insulation is too high, the heat is not dissipated quickly enough and the temperature rises. This also leads to disturbances in the night's sleep – as anyone who has ever been unable to sleep during a hot summer's night knows.

A good sleep system ensures that it doesn't get too cold in winter (so that you don't lose too much heat) or too hot in summer (so that you release sufficient heat to the environment). Because of this, we also strive to maintain a fairly constant body temperature overnight. Incidentally, this is lower during the night than during the day: on average it falls by 1.8 to 2.7°F. There are also small temperature differences between REM and Non-REM sleep. Research has shown that good sleepers generally have a slightly lower body temperature and deeper sleep at night than poor sleepers (Figure 33).

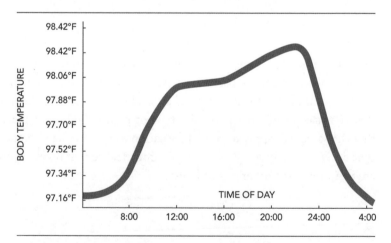

Figure 33   Fluctuations in body temperature of an adult during a day.

Apart from body temperature, there are other important heat variables during a night's sleep: the temperature of the environment, the surface temperature, the bed temperature and the skin temperature, to name only a few.

The normal bed temperature, measured between the body and the duvet, fluctuates between 89.6 and 93.2°F. If a bed does not dissipate excess heat sufficiently, the temperature can rise by up to 1.8°F per hour. This can significantly reduce the proportion of deep sleep in our nightly cycle.

When we are awake, the average temperature of the surface of our skin at the level of our trunk varies between 82.4 and 91.4°F. Usually the temperature rises during the night's rest to a fairly constant 93.2 to 95°F (Figure 34).

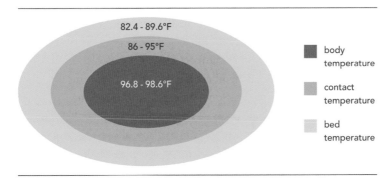

Figure 34   Optimal temperature of a healthy microclimate.

Figure 35 indicates that the skin temperature is stabilised after about 25 minutes, at least in someone sleeping on a sleep system with a good thermal insulation. What we must certainly avoid is that the skin temperature exceeds 96.8°F, because then our body initiates a feedback process that can seriously disrupt our sleep. In Chapter 11, we will discuss that more extensively.

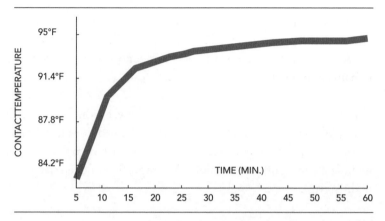

Figure 35   Average contact temperature relative to the sleeping time.

To a large extent, the core of the mattress determines the thermal insulation capability of the sleep system. Foam and latex cores, for instance, have a higher thermal insulation than mattresses with an innerspring core.

The outer cover of the mattress also plays a role. This is usually quilted with a filling. If the fibers are capable of retaining the air well, they will insulate better. Stationary air is one of the strongest insulators.

In addition, the bed linen – sheets, duvet, pillows – also convey heat to the surroundings. More information about this will follow in Chapter 10. For now, it is sufficient to understand that if we want a good night's sleep, we ought to keep our body temperature within a certain range. Unfortunately, a number of factors are complicating this.

First of all, we might live in a climate with significant temperature differences between winter and summer. In newer, well-insulated houses, those temperature differences are smaller, but in older houses, the difference between winter and summer temperatures can vary quite a bit. The conclusion is that a sleep system with a high heat insulation can serve perfectly in the cold months, but is inadequate in the warmer periods because it cannot dissipate the additional heat. Therefore, we must ensure that our sleep system has a wide heat range – so it can cope with these divergent situations. The right duvet is important as well.

Also, the ideal bedroom temperature is 64.4°F, but the temperature of the bed is actually more important. We can influence that by choosing the right sleep system – the right mattress, the right bed base, the right bed linen.

✕ Tip

If you have it too hot at night, you can choose to cover up with a duvet filled with cotton, silk or light down. For cold nights, we recommend a winter down duvet: it weighs very little, falls nicely around your body, absorbs and dissipates a lot of moisture, and has excellent insulating properties. Nowadays there exist special synthetic duvets with similar characteristics. We would suggest to go to a specialized bed store for this.

Partners who sleep together might each need a different kind of heat regulation – one might prefer to sleep warmer than the other – although they still share the same sleep system.

In such cases, sleeping on two separate mattresses might be the option. Anyone who likes sleeping warmer should choose a highly insulating latex mattress. The heat generators among us may prefer a innerspring mattress, because that dissipates the hot air more quickly. You can get good advice on this in a specialized bed store. Customized bed linen could partially compensate for those preference differences.

MOISTURE REGULATION

Our body emits on average 1.35 to 2.02 ounces of water per hour to the surroundings – roughly equivalent to a quarter of a small bottle of soft drink. We lose about one third through our breathing system, the remainder through our body surface.

This adds up to about 6.76 to 10.14 ounces of moisture a night. For some people this can be more than 33.81 ounces or even 84.93 ounces a night. You can easily find out how much moisture you emit by weighing yourself before you go to sleep, and again first thing in the morning. The difference is the weight of the moisture that you've discharged overnight.

For a proper understanding: here we are talking about the moisture that we evaporate unnoticed every hour of every day through exhalation and light perspiration through the skin, even when it is very cold. Anyone who sweats profusely during a hot or feverish night will lose far more moisture. Every drop of moisture that our body loses contains dissolved salts, ballast and harmful substances. About three quarters of it is dissipated through the duvet and the gaps between the duvet, the body and the mattress. The remainder, one quarter, must be dissipated through the mattress and the bed base.

The relative humidity measured between the skin and the sleep system should not become too high. If this nonetheless occurs, then the bed will feel clammy and moist, which is not conducive to sleep. With a good sleep system, the degree of relative humidity between skin and sleep system will be stabilized after about 20 to 25 minutes (Figure 36).

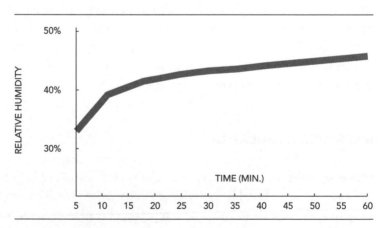

Figure 36   Average relative humidity relative to the sleeping time.

CHAPTER 4

So the mattress and the bed linen must absorb the moisture that we evaporate without leaving a feeling of clamminess, and at the same time it must be able to exchange moisture with the air. Otherwise, all that dampness would simply pass through the mattress and condense at the bottom of the mattress, what could lead to mold formation.

Regulation of humidity has nothing to do with personal preference. The rule is simple: the more moisture the sleep system can absorb and transport, the better. In case of the mattress, the cover constitutes the first moisture buffer – people who sweat a lot at night can opt for a cover and filling that are suitable to perform those tasks as efficiently as possible.

To air the mattress in the morning and let it dry also helps. It might be a good idea to heat the room, because warm air absorbs more moisture than cold air. The disadvantage of heating the room is that afterwards you should air the room, which could cause your energy bill to go up considerably.

It is advisable to air out the bed linen throughout the day and only to make up the bed just before bedtime. Airing out for ten or fifteen minutes is not enough, because the heat and humidity from the bed cannot be adequately dissipated during such a short time – and heat and humidity is what house dust mites are so fond of. Also using a mattress protector as well as a fitted sheet of 100 percent cotton is advisable – cotton has very good moisture regulating properties. Refresh the mattress protector, sheets and duvet covers weekly.

If you have a mattress that you can turn over, certainly do that regularly – at least four times a year. This improves a lower moisture load, prolongs the lifetime of the mattress and prevents a one-sided pressure indentation. If the mattress has symmetrical comfort zones, they can be turned over in the longitudinal direction.

WHAT SHOULD ONE LOOK FOR WHEN BUYING A BED?

We have listed a few important practical conditions that a good bed should meet. Some will seem quite obvious, but it is amazing how often they are overlooked.

- ✕ **Manageability:** All parts of the bed should be easily accessible. It should be easy to make the bed, air it out and maintain it. Cleaning and vacuuming under the bed are also part of this.
- ✕ **Stability:** A sleep system must be stable so you can easily get in and out of bed and you can turn smoothly while lying down. A bed should not sag too much or rock afterwards if you change position.
- ✕ **Sturdiness:** Applies particularly to the bed base. It must be able to cope with the weight of a sleeper who could wearily plop down on his bed late at night.
- ✕ **Durability:** Mattresses are constantly put under pressure. As a result, they will wear out. Even if they are of good quality, they will be 1 to 15 percent less comfortable after ten years. This is the time to buy a new one! Durability is partly determined by external

factors. Someone who perspires a lot and does not ventilate his bed well, will need a new mattress sooner. Sleeping in a damp room also shortens the life of the mattress. Generally, there is a clear link between the price and the durability of a sleep system.

BED COMFORT

A bed must be big enough to allow us to safely change position during sleep.

Length

A bed should ideally be at least 8 to 12 inches longer than the sleeper – a length of 80 inches is consequently a good size for most people. You must be able to lie stretched out on your back in a bed, with having some extra space at the head for a pillow – those 8 inches which we calculated to be added to the body height are by no means an unnecessary luxury.

Width

A bed should at least be wide enough for you to fit in lying on your side with your knees bent. For someone with long legs an amount of space of 40 inches could be necessary. Various studies show that a width of 35 inches is usually enough to sleep comfortably – so for a double bed about 70 inches is needed. Of course, we must take into account individual factors: not everyone has the same width measurement, and anyone who tosses and turns a lot will also need more space.

The width of the mattress will depend on several factors such as body weight, tendency to perspiration (a wider mattress will be able to dissipate more moisture), shoulder width.

Height

Low beds may look beautiful, but they put a lot of strain on the back of whoever makes up the bed and whoever has to get in and out.

The rule of thumb is that the distance between the edge of the mattress and the floor must be at least 18 inches. A really comfortable bed height is when the edge of the mattress is a few inches above the crook of the knee when standing upright. A good bed height is roughly equivalent to a proper sitting height.

Beds with a height of 22 to 24 inches make it easier to stand up from the bed and sit down. A high bed is especially recommended for older people and people with disabilities. Making up the bed is easier, and cleaning around it will take less effort.

Furthermore, it is best to keep a space of 8 inches between the bed and the floor. So you don't have to bend down too low while vacuuming or mopping.

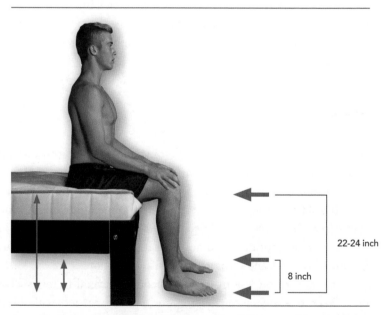

22-24 inch

8 inch

Figure 37 Beds with a height of 22 to 24 inches make it easier to stand up and sit down.

ADJUSTABLE SLEEP SYSTEMS

As we talk about bed comfort, we would like to elaborate on an adjustable bed base. An adjustable bed base has hinges that permits the raising and lowering of the backrest and the head and/or foot ends. This increases the functionality and comfort of the bed, and could also be of great help medically. Some beds have to be adjusted by hand, others have an electric motor that drives the hinges.

Research shows that we don't just sleep in our bed: 16 percent of the time we love to hang out in bed (for example, watching TV), 17 percent of the time we spend reading and 5 percent we use a bed for exercises, etc. So in total we are spending only 62 percent of our time in the bedroom sleeping. Currently this percentage is also changing because of increasing use of media in the bedroom. As to the other activities, it may indeed be useful to be able to adjust the bed. We will now look at a few positions that an adjustable bed facilitates.

Flat lying position

The user is asleep or taken care of.

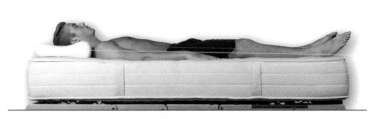

Figure 38   Sleeping flat.

Feet elevated

This gives the feet extra rest, which can be very useful for varicose veins or oedema in the legs.

Raising the foot end also stimulates the blood circulation, because the blood flows back to the heart more easily (Figure 39), which in turn improves the quality of sleep. A continuous slight elevation of two to three degrees will form no problem. A higher elevation can be especially useful for short breaks during the day. Make sure that the high settings of the bed run over the full length of the bed when you go to sleep. Otherwise you will end up with bending points causing your pelvis to tilt. (Figures 40 and 41).

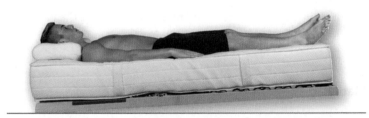

Figure 39   Sleep correction over the full lying length promotes the return of the blood through the veins.

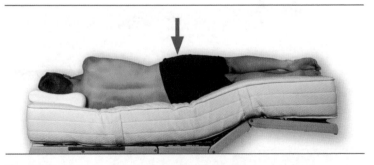

Figure 40   Incorrect use of bending points can cause back pain.

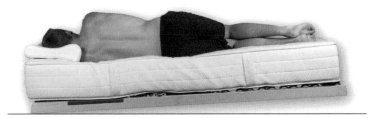

Figure 41 A sleep correction over the full lying length ensures correct support of the spinal column.

Half-sitting position with knee support

Sleeping or resting in this position may be more comfortable or even necessary for some people, for instance when having a respiratory problem.

The angled adjustments of the bed base should counteract the shifts of the body. The optimal settings are shown in Figure 42. For a comfortable sleep, the angle between the horizontal plane and the back rest should not exceed 40 degrees.

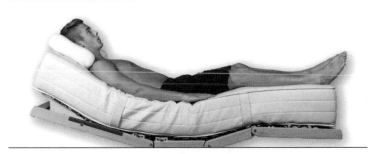

Figure 42 Resting in a half-sitting position with knee support.

Sitting position

This position is useful for someone carrying out activities in bed, such as talking, reading, eating and drinking, etc. This is also a good starting position for getting in and out of bed. The angle of adjustment should again counteract movements of the body. The optimal setting is shown in Figure 43. An adjustable headrest can increase comfort. Reading in bed during the day is best done in this position and not in a half-sitting position without knee support, because in this position, the back can be bent in the same way as in a poor sitting position. If you then slide further down, the risk of back pain increases (Figure 44).

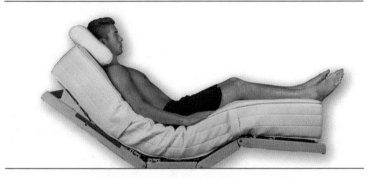

Figure 43   Good sitting and reading position with head and knee support.

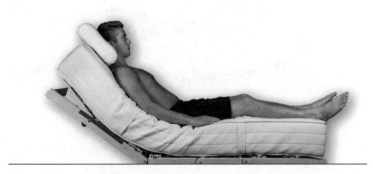

Figure 44   Poor sitting position with increased risk of sliding down and back pain.

The half-sitting position without knee support also encourages bed-sores in the case of bedridden patients. You are no longer sitting on your sit bones, but on the sacrum, making the bottom capable of sliding down on the mattress. This will cause frictional forces, which can lead to blood circulation problems and bedsores. This position can also cause bedsores on the heels, because you will plant your heels firmly into the mattress to prevent sliding down.

We can minimise those shifts by fully tilting the bed. As a result, the body's centre of gravity moves backwards and you will be less prone to sliding down (Figure 45).

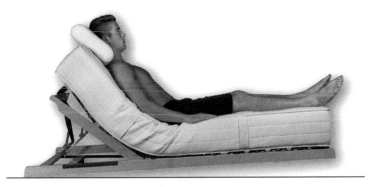

Figure 45   Comfortable sitting position with less chance of sliding down.

A motorized adjustable bed can also help patients or the elderly to sit up straight in bed: first raise the thigh support and then the back-rest. This way, you minimize sliding on to the mattress and the base (Figure 46). To get out of the bed from a sitting position you lower the foot section. If you're going back to sleep, repeat these movements in reverse order.

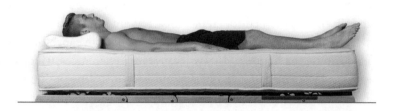

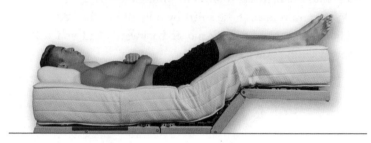

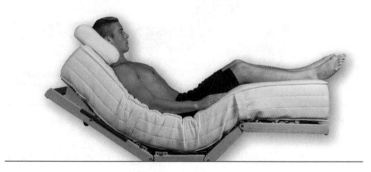

Figure 46

74

Hard versus soft

We learned already a great deal. We now know how the spinal column is put together, how lower back pain occurs and how this influences sleep problems, and what conditions a good bed must meet. In this chapter we will examine what effect our sleep system can have on the health of our back. We're going to do this using one of the basic facts about beds, of which many misunderstandings exist, namely hard versus soft sleep surfaces.

If your bed base or mattress is too soft and sags too much, your body – and thus also your spinal column – will bend along with it. When lying on your side, your spinal column will no longer form a straight line, but will be bent like a banana. This will cause also additional problems: your range of movement will be reduced, and your moisture regulation will be less efficient.

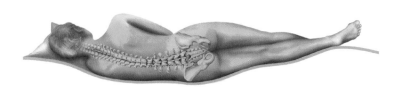

Figure 47   The hammock effect with a sleep system that is too soft has a negative influence on the spinal column.

In a sleep system that is **too soft**, it is as if your body is lying in a dip. We call this the *hammock effect*. Often, when this happens, people will place a board on the sagging bed base as an emergency solution. This is not a good idea, because then the mattress has to carry out two functions: that of a good, resilient, but also supportive bed base and that of the mattress. As a result, it will never be able to guarantee optimum comfort.

If you leave the board in place for a longer period, the chance of growing mold on the underside of the mattress will increase.

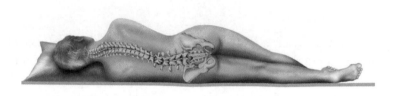

Figure 48   A sleep system that is too hard has a negative influence on the spinal column as well.

If you are sleeping on a sleep system that is **too hard**, you will get a very different problem: the spinal column will distort, particularly when lying on your side – the dominant sleep position. The pressure on the skin and underlying tissues is greatly increased, and you will change position more frequently, which takes a lot of energy.

Both sleep systems, that are too soft and too hard, will reduce the quality of sleep and may lead to pain symptoms. The trick is to choose a sleep system that suits you. As always, it's down to finding the middle way. To illustrate the symptoms to which a sleep system that is too hard or too soft leads, we will relate the experiences of two patients. But to be able to understand their story properly, we first need to explain a bit more about our pain mechanism.

CUTTING OR GNAWING PAIN?

There are sensors in our body that inform us about tissue damage or threats that can lead to tissue damage. The signal that they use for that message is one we all know: *pain.*

CHAPTER 5

Pain is a protection mechanism: as soon as the sensors convey to our brain that something is wrong, the body will try to escape that threat. Hold a finger over the flame of a candle and you will immediately know what we mean by this. Figure 49 shows a (simplified) schematic representation of the course of the sensory nerve from the skin to the brain.

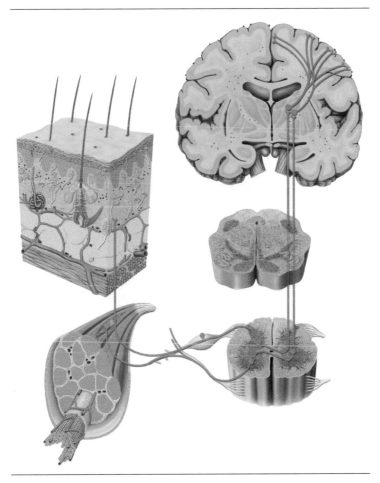

Figure 49 Schematic representation of the course of a stimulus (for instance pain, temperature, coarse touch). The stimulus departs the skin (blue line) towards the brain, which sends feedback to the muscle fibers (red line).

There are many pain sensors in our skin and fewer in deeper-lying structures such as muscles, blood vessels and joints. At the level of the epidermis, there are sensitive nerve endings, fine touch and pressure sensors and cold and heat receptors (see Figure 50).

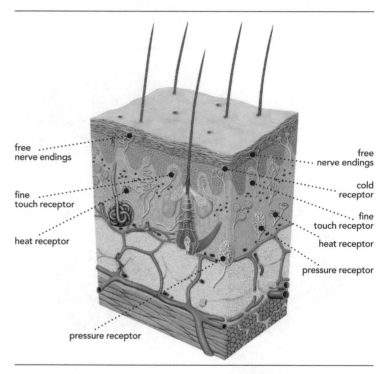

Figure 50 Cross-section of the skin with its main free nerve endings, fine touch and pressure sensors, and cold and heat receptors.

That's why, for the most part, we perceive a pain stimulus in our epidermis as fierce, sharp and cutting. We can also accurately locate this pain, and it usually disappears after a while. However, if pain comes from a deeper level, it is generally crushing, gnawing and more difficult to delineate. Sometimes it even radiates to totally different parts of the body, for instance you will feel pain in your leg while the cause might be a hernia.

We can only measure the pain intensity subjectively. Patients can usually give a good description of what the pain feels like: crushing and gnawing, or fierce and cutting. From this description we can learn a lot about the underlying causes.

We will now look more closely at two patients with symptoms that are typical for non-specific lower back pain and we will look into what we can deduct from their story about their sleep system. Quite a lot, as it turns out.

PATIENT 1: MALE, AGE 40, REGULAR BODY SHAPE

'Every morning, I get up with lower back pain, which gradually disappears. The pain is burning, and my lower back muscles are stiff, as if I've played hard at sports. The sore spot also feels heavy. I am able to fall asleep at night, but every so often I wake up because of pain. In the morning, I don't feel very fit.'

The pain that our first patient is talking about is more than likely the result of prolonged burdening of soft tissue such as ligaments and joint capsules. The burdening is the result of incorrect support of the spinal column. The cause could be a sleep system that is too soft.

If we repeatedly put pressure on the soft tissue every night, the pain sensors can become less sensitive. As a result, the brain will not receive a timely signal of impending tissue damage. The body remains in the same position of burdening for too long and the ligaments and joint capsules become damaged. This leads to that heavy feeling and the feeling of muscle stiffness that this patient is talking about.

PATIENT 2: FEMALE, AGE 60, REGULAR BODY SHAPE

'I can't find a comfortable position to fall asleep in, I lie tossing and turning all night, and in the morning I get up with lower back pain. My shoulders and neck also feel very stiff. I go to bed early, and I lie in bed for seven to eight hours, but I still don't feel fully rested. I wake up a couple of times during the night.'

The symptoms of our second patient are typical of someone who has a sleep system that is too hard. To begin with, she has difficulty falling asleep because she is lying on top of the mattress. The sleep system doesn't yield at the points of her body on which her weight rests. Those points come under great pressure, which feels unpleasant or painful. Finding a comfortable position in which to fall asleep isn't possible.

If she is able to grab some sleep, the high pressure on the skin surface persists. That pressure can penetrate to the muscle and fatty tissue and pinch off the blood vessels, resulting in a local lack of oxygen. When this is detected by the brain, the brain sends out a signal to change position, so that the blood circulation resumes. That means that this patient will be lying tossing and turning at night. Figure 51 shows the main pressure points for lying on your back and side. All of the pressure points are located at the level of bony protrusions, where the layer of fat is much thinner than elsewhere in the body and where there are no thick muscle layers capable of distributing the forces.

When we sleep, the tension in our muscles decreases. When we are lying on a system that is too hard, the spinal column segments will deflect into an unnatural position because of that decreased muscle tension. Soft tissue such as ligaments, muscles, inter-vertebral discs, joint capsules, nerve tissue and bone structures are put under tension, which may initiate pain symptoms such as lower back pain and stiffness in the neck and shoulders.

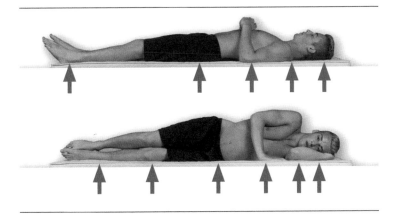

Figure 51   The locations of pressure-sensitive zones in supine and lateral positions.

We are not sure if people who sleep on a system that is too hard get enough deep sleep. They will reach their seven or eight hours of sleep, but their sleep quality will be poor. Lying in your bed for a long time is certainly no guarantee of a good night's sleep.

POSITIONS IN A SLEEP SYSTEM THAT IS TOO SOFT

Now that we know the general principle of sleep systems that are too hard or too soft, we can become more specific. What are the consequences of a sleep system that is too soft for people who sleep on their back, side or stomach?

Supine position (lying on your back)

If you are sleeping on your back in a bed that is too soft, your spinal column will sag completely. The pelvis usually tilts backwards, and the legs end up lying a little bit higher. This leads to a flexion in the hip joint. This bending of the hip results in a reduced pull on the iliopsoas or internal hip flexor. As a result, the natural curve of the spinal column at the level of the waist is reduced. It's just like lying in a hammock.

As we pointed out in Chapter 2, **bending** of the spinal column has consequences for the facet joints, inter-vertebral discs and all soft tissue – ligaments, muscles, nerves – of the motion segment.

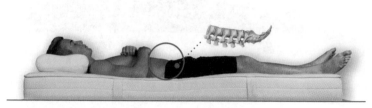

Figure 52   The lower back vertebrae sag completely as in flexion.

Prone position (lying on your belly)

Sleeping on your stomach on a soft support surface creates in turn a **stretching** of the spinal column. This will mostly put a strain on the facet joints. Moreover, you will have to turn your head to breath. As a result, your spinal column undergoes a rotational movement, which leads to a rotational strain on the facet joints, ligaments, inter-vertebral discs, muscles – in a nutshell, on all the structures of the motion segment.

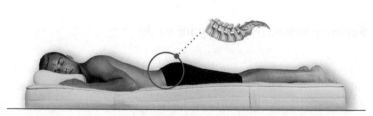

Figure 53   The facet joints at the level of the lower back are overloaded as in an extension movement.

82

Lateral position (lying on your side)

In the lateral position, the pelvis sags too much because the pelvis is the heaviest point of the body. At the top of the spinal column, the facet joints and inter-vertebral discs will be compressed and at the bottom, soft tissue structures such as joint capsules and ligaments will come under tension.

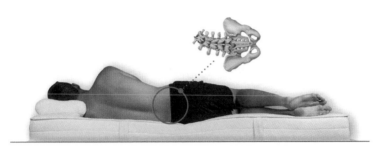

Figure 54   The lumbar vertebrae sag, as in a lateral movement, and deviate from the desired horizontal line.

POSITIONS IN A SLEEP SYSTEM THAT IS TOO HARD

Lateral position (lying on your side)

When we lie on our side, a sleep system that is too hard will primarily support our shoulders and our pelvis, while the lumbar spine sags and the back, when viewed from behind, will exhibit an unnatural S-shaped curve (Figure 55).

This is because our shoulders are broader than our hips and our waist is narrower than both the hips and the shoulders. Under the influence of gravity and the reduced nocturnal muscle tension, the lumbar vertebrae will sag too. In this situation, the spinal column can be compared with a suspension bridge secured at two points of support:

shoulder and pelvis. There are four bending points: at the shoulders, the pelvis, in the middle of the lower back (the lowest point of the suspension bridge), and at the transition from the neck to the thoracic vertebrae. All movement segments come under an uneven load, so that the nucleus of the inter-vertebral disc will shift.

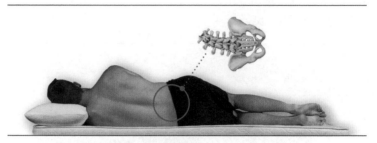

Figure 55 All the vertebrae are unevenly loaded and exhibit an S-shaped curve. The lumbar vertebrae will also deflect, as in a lateral movement.

Supine position (lying on your back)

It is not certain what sleeping on our back on a hard system means for our spinal column. Furter research about this topic, needs to be conducted. But we can assume that the curves of the spinal column will level off because of the decreased muscle tension and the backward tilt of the pelvis. The lower back would also sag slightly, but that distortion would be less extreme than when we sleep on a soft system.

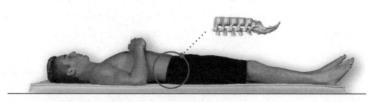

Figure 56 The lumbar vertebrae will in all probability sag and the spinal column curvatures will lessen.

Prone position (lying on your stomach)

Not much is known about sleeping on your belly on a hard system. We can assume that the lumbar curve flattens out – to what extent will depend on the abdominal volume of the sleeper.

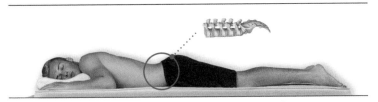

Figure 57   The lumbar vertebrae will in all probability be flattened, but this is also highly dependent on the abdominal volume.

Barely 5 to 10 percent of all people persistently sleep on their stomach. Usually, those people move in the course of the night to a semi-prone/semi-lateral position. Unfortunately, because of the rotation of the head, a lot of tension in the cervical spine will arise.

THE DAMAGE

Therefore we may conclude that sleep systems that are too hard or too soft are not good for the back. Both systems will distort our spinal column. That will put all the structures around the spinal column, the shoulders and the pelvis under pressure, and can lead to the complaints discussed in Chapter 2: non-specific lower back pain.

CHANGES IN POSITION

We often change position during our sleep. So it is important that our bed gives us freedom of range of movement, and that it supports our body enough to be able to move in a relaxed way.

The resilience of our sleep system is very important here. It must yield very quickly where needed, for instance at the shoulders and the hips. It must also quickly bounce back when we shift our body, otherwise the body is not well supported and it cannot remain lying in a stable condition. Especially for patients with back pain is this a very important factor.

It is normal and even necessary that we change positions frequently. If we were to lie in the same position for a longer time, we would put continuously strain on certain body structures, which is obviously not a good idea. By changing positions, we will disperse this pressure.

Continuously shifting to another position, on the other hand, is not ideal. By moving too often we consume energy at a time when we should rest. We also need to make sure we have enough deep sleep stages at night; otherwise we will not feel fresh the next day.

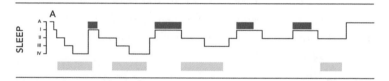

Figure 58 Postural immobility (pink blocks) in relation to the sleep cycle. The EEG data are shown as follows: wakefulness (A), non-REM phases I, II, III, IV and REM sleep (red blocks).

During Non-REM sleep, especially during our deep sleep, we have fairly long periods in which we do not move – according to some researchers between 45 to 75 minutes (see Figure 58). Formerly, it was supposed that there was a link between how often we change position and our sleep quality, but recent research refutes that hypothesis. There appears to be big differences among people with regard to the number of changes of position – too big a number to be able to draw general conclusions. The proportion of deep sleep appears to be an important indicator of the quality of sleep.

We will now take a look at the influence of sleep systems that are too soft or too hard on changes of position.

Too soft

In a sleep system that is too soft, your body will sag too deeply in the mattress and you risk that the mattress will enclose your body too much. That makes it more difficult to change position because you will have to push yourself up sideways. You will always end up in 'the hammock' no matter what you do. Your body will keep looking for a good position, which costs energy and reduces sleep quality. Also be cautious for sleeping on mattresses that have too much viscoelastic (memory) foam. More explanation will follow in chapter 6.

Back pain patients who sleep on a soft system often ask for a mattress that is as firm as possible because they are afraid of sinking into the mattress too deeply – they want stable support. But actually, they don't mean a firm mattress so much as a stable mattress, one that doesn't wobble too much after movement and certainly doesn't sag like a hammock. Lying on something a bit too hard is certainly not good, but better than lying on something too soft.

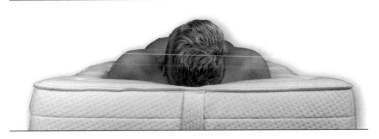

Figure 59 A mattress that is too soft encloses your body too much and that hampers smooth changing of position.

Too hard

If you are sleeping on a sleep system that is too hard, you will move too easily, because the mattress surrounds your body insufficiently. Assuming a stable body position is more difficult because there are too few contact points. The pressure on those contact points is also uncomfortably high.

Obese people will be less disadvantaged by sleep systems that are too hard, because the body fat acts as a kind of cushion. They often have less defined body contours when reclining and they have a larger contact surface with the sleep system. The pressure is no longer concentrated at a few points, but is distributed.

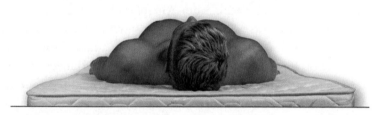

Figure 60 A mattress that is too firm will not enclose your body enough: it is as if you are lying 'on top of' the mattress.

MOISTURE AND HEAT REGULATION

It may sound strange at first, but a sleep system that is too soft or too hard also has a negative effect on moisture and heat regulation.

Too soft

When we lie on a mattress that is too soft, a greater proportion of our body makes contact with the sleep system. The relative humidity is higher at that contact surface, because we dissipate moisture less easily to the sleep system than to the air. At the same time, a smaller part of the skin is exposed to the air. The end result: the mattress needs to dissipate more moisture.

This is no easy task and the probability is high that the bed climate will become more humid and warmer and skin contact temperature will rapidly rise to above 95°F. This is fatal to a good night's rest.

Too hard

We still know too little about the impact of sleeping on too hard a surface regarding moisture and heat regulation. It seems logical that the smaller contact surface will lead to reduced thermal insulation, resulting in a lower bed and skin temperature, but we will have to wait for the results of more research before we can pass a decisive judgment on that.

Mattresses and bed bases

In the Western world, we hardly used to think about a good bed. People slept on straw mattresses, and later on sagging mattresses and saggy springs. Suddenly, in the 1950s, sleeping on a hard bed base was promoted as a remedy for back pain. Waterbeds and soft sleep systems were a hype in the eighties. Nowadays, we take a much more nuanced approach to sleep systems and distinguish three main components: the mattress, bed base or foundation, and the pillow.

Additionally, there is the bed frame, the furniture that supports the sleep system. Of course, this has to be sufficiently solid but otherwise has it no effect on the sleep comfort. Nowadays you also have the posibility of putting your bed base freestanding on legs.

MATTRESSES

From the outside, mattresses all look more or less alike, but there are very big differences with regard to the outer fabric, the surface fillings in the covers or the inside structure (or mattress core construction). A mattress consists of a core, possibly one or more covering layers (made of upholstery materials and also called comfort layers), and a cover. The thickness varies from about 6 to more than 11 inches. Let's take a thorough look at the inner structure of the mattress types.

There are three main types: foam, latex and innerspring mattresses. In addition, there are less common types such as air, gel or water mattresses.

Foam mattresses

The core of a foam mattress consists of one large block of foam. We will explain what foam looks like and what types of foam mattresses are on the market, but first we will enumerate the factors that determine the quality of the mattress.

» Density

Density is a measurement of mass per unit of volume. It is primarily the durability of foam mattresses that is determined by it. The higher the density, the longer they will last. Density generally ranges between 2lbs all the way up to over 7lbs/cubic feet. This makes sense, because the more material used, the more forces can be absorbed.

» Firmness

A second important feature is the firmness. There is a special relationship between density and firmness: the lower the density of the foam, the more rapidly loss of firmness occurs. This implies that dips in the mattress will form more quickly and that it will wear out faster.

Now, in foam mattresses, firmness is partly linked to the density: a soft mattress with low density will wear out faster. Fortunately, the firmness also depends partly on the type of foam. Nowadays, manufacturers are able to produce foam mattresses with a high density that are nonetheless soft enough to ensure good conformity and pressure distribution (Figure 61).

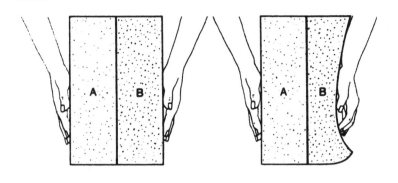

Figure 61   Foams A and B have the same density but different firmness.
Foam B is softer than foam A.

» Elasticity

Elasticity or resilience is one of the most important properties of a mattress. When laying down, the mattress should immediately deform according to the conformity principle. Protruding parts of your body such as shoulders and hips should be able to partially sink in. Receding portions, such as the waist in many women, should be supported. Elasticity can be described as the speed and efficiency with which that happens. A mattress with good elasticity and high flexibility will therefore respond immediately and give you the appropriate support if you change your position.

Elasticity and flexibility also determine the extent to which two people can lie next to each other without either noticing the movements of the other. If you feel movement whenever your partner turns around, your mattress is not that good.

The mattress industry speaks of two types of elasticity: *surface elasticity* and *point elasticity*. Surface elasticity means: a large part of the mattress surface deforms under load. The pressure distribution and conformity are not optimal (see Figure 62).

Point elasticity means that a very small part of the mattress surface deforms under load. The pressure distribution and conformity are much better.

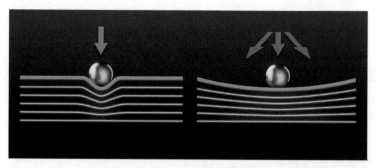

Figurre 62 With point elasticity (left), a small area deforms under load and the material springs back quickly. With surface elasticity (right), on the other hand, a large area deforms under load.

You can easily try out both types of elasticity at home. Make a solid fist and give it a shove into your mattress and see how far the area around your fist deforms. Then quickly pull back your fist and see to what extent the deformed material springs back quickly. A local deformation and rapid recovery of the deformed material is good.

Air passage plays a role in the elasticity of foam mattresses. When you lie down, you push the air in the mattress away from you. If you change your position, the air returns to the places where you are no longer exerting any pressure, and the air flows away from the places where you are now exerting force. A mattress breathes. Tests have shown that the elasticity of a foam mattress increases as the air circulates through it more easily.

Foam mattresses with a high density and variable firmness generally have a good elasticity.

» Heat and moisture regulation

Foam mattresses are always more insulating than innerspring mattresses. This is great for people who feel a bit chilly in bed. For someone who feels easily too hot an innerspring mattress might be better suited.

We cannot make general statements about the moisture regulation of foam mattresses. This depends too much on the quality of the mattress.

» Types of foam

✕ Polyether

Polyether is a synthetic foam that is made up of millions of cells. Mattresses with polyether foam have a good thermal insulation, but moderate moisture permeation and conformity. Because of the light weight they are easy to handle.

The minimum thickness of a mattress made of reasonable quality foam is 6 inches. The density must be at least 1.8lbs/cubic feet. The higher the density, the longer the life of the mattress will be. Polyether foam exists in firmer and softer versions.

✕ HR foam

These foams are also made up of millions of microscopically small cells. They are non-allergenic, odourless and contain no heavy metals. The production is completely CFC-free. They have a higher density and better conformity than the traditional polyether foams.

HR stands for High Resilience. The material has a somewhat irregular, open cell structure, with the result that it breathes well and dissipates moisture better.

HR foam mattresses with a thickness of between 6 and 10 inches with comfort zones and well-suited density belong to the better foam mattresses.

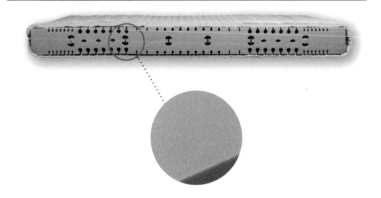

Figure 63 HR foam mattress with comfort zones. The foam structure is very comparable to that of a sponge.

× Viscoelastic foam

Viscoelastic foam, also called slow recovery foam, slow pressure-relief foam, NASA foam, lazy foam or, as it is almost universally called in the UK and US, memory foam. The sleeper's body heat and weight will soften it. When you push viscoelastic foam in, it will flow away from you, without a definite end point. That's where the name has its origin: elastic refers to the deformability of this material; visco to the fluidity.

This is the most controversial material in the European and American mattress industry.

Foam that relieves too much to pressure is bad for conformity because it does not adequately support the spinal column. It might be very useful for patients with an increased risk of pressure sores.

The foam reacts slowly: after being squashed, it takes 0.5 to 5 seconds to return to its original shape. It is thus much less resilient than HR foam and latex mattresses. Changing positions when asleep will not happen very smoothly, which reduces the sleep quality.

This foam may also feel hard in a cool environment and very soft in a warm environment. The better viscoelastic foams are actually less temperature dependent and some also spring back faster after loading.

In general, we can state: with an equal density, HR foam has better comfort features than viscoelastic foam, especially when it comes to conformity and elasticity.

Viscoelastic foam is usually used as a thin covering layer on top of HR foam or pocket spring mattresses.

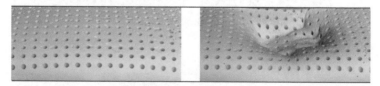

Figure 64   Viscoelastic foam deforms locally under load, but springs back slowly, hence the name slow recovery foam.

Latex mattresses

Latex mattresses or rubber mattresses consist of small, foamed rubber particles. Mattresses may consist of synthetic latex, natural latex from the *Hevea brasiliensis* tree, or a blend of both. The production process is comparable to baking waffles: a fluidity, lightly whipped material is poured into a mold and baked. This process dates back to 1839, and was invented by Charles Goodyear.

» Synthetic and natural latex

Natural latex is made from the sap of the rubber tree. Car tires and condoms are also made of this material. A natural latex mattress is made up of 50 to 95 percent natural rubber, in addition to other substances, inter alia to keep the material permanently elastic.

Mattresses with a high content of natural latex are more elastic than those which consist primarily of synthetic latex. These mattresses adjust themselves really well to the load exerted on them, and score very well in terms of conformity and pressure distribution (see Figure 65). However, they are relatively heavy.

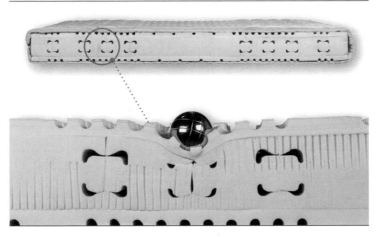

Figure 65   High-conforming latex mattress with comfort zones.

Synthetic latex is a petroleum product. Mattresses consisting of 100 percent synthetic latex are less comfortable than natural latex mattresses. All latex mattresses have a higher density than most synthetic foams.

» Thermal insulation, moisture regulation and conformity

Latex has a structure that ensures a constant air circulation (Figure 66). Often, the manufacturer makes additional horizontal ventilation holes in the mattress. If you move during your sleep, a kind of pump effect is created which allows for good air circulation. Latex mattresses have a good conformity. They have good heat insulation and are sufficiently permeable to moisture.

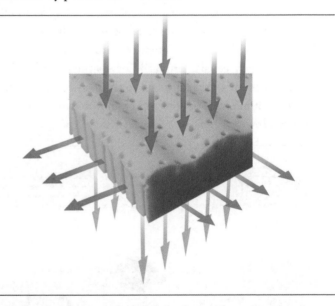

Figure 66 Latex has microscopically small air chambers which ensure good air circulation.

Innerspring mattresses

Innerspring mattresses are among the 'classics' when it comes to mattresses. It is already in the name: the core of an innerspring mattress consists of a large number of mutually connected steel springs. The comfort of a spring core is highly dependent on the ultimate construction and, among other factors, the shape, height, diameter and wire thickness of the springs (wire gauge). The innerspring is covered with padding or upholstery materials, which can include various foams, latex, fiber, and additional layers of smaller steel springs. These are often referred to as the 'comfort layers'. If an innerspring core is combined with high-end polyurethane foams or latex as a comfort layer, it is sometimes called a 'Hybrid Bed'.

The spring constructions can be divided into two large groups: open coil springs and pocket springs.

» Open coil springs

The most widely used option is the Bonnell spring. Bonnell springs are knotted, round-top, hourglass-shaped steel wire coils. When laced together with cross wire helicals, these coils form the simplest innerspring unit, also referred to as a Bonnell unit. The Bonnell springs have a 'narrowed waist' shape like an hourglass and are wider at the ends than in the middle (see Figure 67).

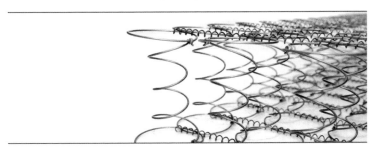

Figure 67 Bonnell springs are wider at top and bottom and are interconnected with each other by a spiral wire.

Bonnell springs are, for stability, arranged in rows and connected to one another, at the top and at the bottom, by means of a spiral helical wire and with an outer rod strengthening the perimeter. Bonnell springs are more rigid than pocket springs. A Bonnell spring mattress has surface elasticity. Over the years, quite a few variations on this technology have been developed. Other well-known open coil springs are the LFK coil and the continuous coil spring unit. LFK coils are an unknotted offset coil with a cylindrical or columnar shape. The continuous spring unit is made from a single length of wire 'knitted' into a series of interwoven springs which usually run up and down the bed and are linked vertically rather than horizontally. The gauge of wires used is softer and the size of the 'coils' is smaller than the Bonnell and LFK units, resulting in a higher spring count and a more responsive feel.

» Pocket springs

Pocket springs, also known as wrapped or encased coils, are thin-gauge, barrel-shaped, knotless coils that are individually encased in fabric pockets. The American engineer John Gail invented them in 1925, and this is still one of the most common mattress technologies in the world. According to several other sources, pocket springs are an invention of James Marshall in 1899, hence the reference to 'Marshall coils'. The number of springs can vary from 200 to more than double that per square metre.

Most springs of this type are cylindrical (equally wide all over) or barrel-shaped (wider in the middle) (see Figure 68). Usually, the springs are aligned in rows. This results in an extremely smooth and flexible mattress core with a high load capacity.

The springs move individually and independently from each other, but they are mutually connected by the fabric pockets being glued together. That makes the mattress stable – a very elegant invention.

Often, the mattress is divided into comfort zones, the firmness of which is controlled by the height of the spring, the position and pre-loading of the spring in the cover, and the thickness of the steel wire. The springs are covered with an insulator pad. On top of that are one or more covering layers, usually made of foam, latex, cotton fiber, wool fiber or polyester fiber. The insulator pad separates the mattress core from the middle upholstery. The quality of those covering layers determines to a large extent the comfort and the longevity of the mattress. These covering layers may be present on one side or on both sides of the pocket core and, in case of foam or latex, the minimum thickness is 1 to 2 inches. If these layers are thinner than 1 inch, then you will easier feel the pocket springs, what of course should not happen. Then it would be advisable to put a topper on top of your mattress. If the pocket spring core has a double-sided finish, you can flip over the mattress two to four times a year.

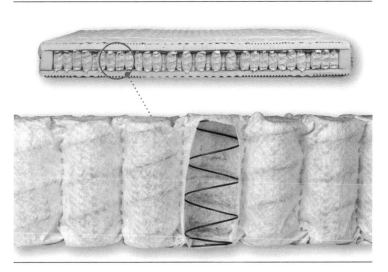

Figures 68 and 69   Pocket spring mattress with comfort zones, covered on both sides with latex.

» Conformity, thermal insulation and moisture regulation

Pocket spring mattresses have a higher point elasticity and therefore a better conformity and pressure distribution than open coil springs (see Figure 70).

Innerspring mattresses have good moisture regulation, that is, if the covering layers and the cover are also made of materials that absorb and dissipate moisture well. With each body movement, air is actually pumped out of the mattress core – thus taking the moisture along with it.

On the other hand, this very same air circulation is also the reason that innerspring mattresses are not scoring so well on thermal insulation. People who quickly feel too warm in bed will be fine with this.

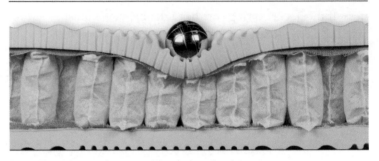

Figure 70   High point elasticity with latex-covered pocket springs.

WATERBED

The waterbed is not included in our survey of sleep systems: it is essentially a hybrid – bed base and mattress in one. Many people who sleep on it never want to change it out for anything else, but it may possibly have some disadvantages for the back. With waterbeds, patients experience the heat as very pleasant.

When sleeping on a waterbed, the heaviest part of the body – the pelvis – will slump deeper than on a regular mattress. As a result, the lower back is poorly supported, which can lead to back pain. Changing the lying position can also be a problem, because there are no stable push-off points. Turning over becomes more difficult, and the extra muscle work you must provide loads the spinal column more than usual. If you already have back problems, the back pain could worsen as a result.

If, for medical reasons (other then back pain), you still want to sleep on a waterbed, it would be best to choose a maximally stabilised dual system: a waterbed with two separate single-person's mattresses with a thickness of approximately 8 inches. This way, your sleep won't be disturbed when your partner turns over, and you can set your own water volume and temperature.

AIRBED

Airbeds use one or more adjustable air chambers as a support system. Unlike the type of air mattresses used for camping, the air chamber of a residential airbed is covered by padding or upholstery materials, which can include various foams and fiber. Some beds of this type are referred to as soft-sided airbeds. Airbeds allow the firmness to be adjusted and usually allow each side of the bed to be controlled separately to meet the individual and changing needs of couples. Airbeds are designed to look like a conventional bed.

COVER AND SURFACE FILLINGS

The first thing you will notice about a mattress is its cover – known in the trade as the ticking. Ticking with special properties is increasingly being used by mattress manufacturers. Some of the options include anti-house dust mite/allergy, antibacterial, antimicrobial, water-resistant, highly absorbent, anti-static etc. The ticking usually consists of a mix of materials, ranging from viscose, cotton, wool, linen or silk to modern synthetic fibers such as polyamide, polyester, microfibers, elastane etc. Knitted mattress fabrics (stretchy knit ticking) are recommended. They are elastic and improve the conformity and pressure distribution of the mattress.

Most mattress covers have three layers: the outer ticking (woven, damask or knitted), the fillings, and the lower fabric backing. Together they form the outer upholstery or cover of the mattress. The cover is a very important part of the mattress. It constitutes the primary moisture and heat regulation and is responsible for a dry sleeping climate.

Most mattresses are finished by either quilting or tufting. Quilting is a decorative effect attaching the outer fabric to the surface fillings; these mattresses tend to have a smoother, flatter surface. Tufting – a process in which tapes are passed right through the mattress at regular intervals and secured on each side by tags or washers – prevents loose filling from being dislodged.

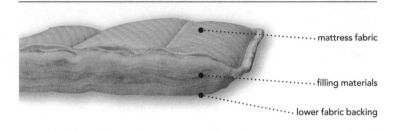

mattress fabric

filling materials

lower fabric backing

Figure 71 The outer cover quilted with filling is a primary moisture buffer for the mattress.

Surface fillings

We will give you a brief overview of the types of surface fillings we frequently encounter in the cover; wool and polyester are used most often.

» Wool

Wool has a strong frizzy, hollow hair structure. As a result, it is very elastic. It is also an excellent thermal insulator because, due to all those curls, it can retain air well. Air, as we know, is an excellent insulator. The use of wool contributes to a comfortable, consistent bed temperature.

Furthermore, it is also a good moisture regulator: it can absorb up to 40 percent of its own weight in vapour without feeling wet. It is the most obvious fiber to use as a filling.

» Cotton

Cotton can absorb up to 28 percent of its own weight in moisture without feeling wet. The thermal insulation properties are less strong, which makes it more of a summer fabric. Usually, part of the mattress cover consists of cotton because it is a very skin-friendly fiber with a strong antibacterial action and is well tolerated by people with an allergy.

» Silk

Silk can absorb up to 30 percent of its own weight in moisture and also dissipates it quickly and easily. As a result, it is great to use in the summer because it's a fiber that is very cool to the touch. Silk hardly insulates at all because it cannot store air. It does therefore have good breathability.

Silk is very suitable for the outer covering of the mattress and is definitely recommended for people who evaporate a lot of moisture or are allergic. Silk is known for its hypoallergenic effect.

» Polyester

Polyester fibers are often used as filling. Manufacturers often endow them with useful properties, such as increased moisture regulation, antibacterial action and so on.

» Acrylics and polyamide

Acrylics and polyamide are also commonly used fillings. They are very elastic, hardly absorb moisture and score less well than wool and silk in the field of thermal insulation. They are combined with wool as a cover filling in better mattresses.

	wool	cotton	silk	polyester	acrylic	polyamide
elasticity	very good	less good	very good	very good	good	good
moisture-absorbing capacity	slowly absorbs a great deal of moisture	quickly absorbs a lot of moisture	easily absorbs a lot of moisture	absorbs very little moisture	absorbs little moisture	absorbs little moisture
thermal insulation	good	less good	good	poor	very good	poor

Figure 72   Elasticity, moisture-absorbing capacity and thermal insulation of the main fillings.

BED BASES

All over the world there are different types of bed bases! Traditions, culture, customs and socio-economic differences play a major role on the available selection or supply in the various parts of the world. In Western Europe especially, slatted bases and box springs are very popular. In the US and the UK, mattresses are more likely to be laid on solid platform beds, box springs or spring edge divans covered with upholstered or wooden headboards, and in the Far East, people sleep on hard sleeping mats.

We provide here a brief overview of the most common bed bases from industrialised countries.

Box springs and divans

Box springs are very popular in Anglo-Saxon countries and this Anglo-American name is a combination of the words 'box' and 'spring'. In other words, this is a rigid frame containing springs. The mattress ultimately lies on top of this. By combining different materials, you get a huge variety of structures and the comfort will greatly depend on the optimum comfort ratio between box and mattress. For the overall combination, various terms are used such as box spring system, box-spring bed. The conformity and hardness of the foundations, or bed bases, depend very much on the structure and quality of the used materials.

The typical box spring has a supporting structure in a wooden frame containing a large number of vertical interior springs. The innersprings may be open coil, but equally, they may be pocket springs. The innerspring is typically covered with a number of top layers, including an insulator pad and foam. Around all this is also a loose cover or ticking.

The spring edge divan has a slightly different structure. In the UK, spring edge divans are very popular. A complete open coil or pocket spring unit is mounted on a wooden frame that acts like a giant shock demper, increasing the mattress's durability.

Box springs and divans are, in essence, upholstered boxes on legs to create space beneath. These days, there are many beautifully tailored and upholstered bases with matching headboards in a range of colors and fabrics on the market.

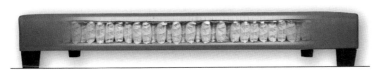

Figure 73   Box spring with pocket springs.

Other constructions are the solid or platform top constructions, having a rigid, non-spring top panel, often made of hardboard or steel. Beds with these bases are generally firmer and are therefore combined with thicker mattresses. Other commonly used names for this are the 'no-flex', 'low-flex' or zero-deflection unit. Both varieties are very popular in the US and the UK.

In Scandinavia, box springs are often the basis of the sleep system. Usually, a spring mattress will be placed upon it, topped with a little mini mattress: the topper. We call that the Scandinavian sleep system.

✗ Topper – Pillow top mattress

Nowadays, there are also mini mattresses – we call those toppers – with an average thickness of 2 to 5 inches. If your mattress meets all comfort requirements, you will not need a topper. Sometimes, however, the topper does constitute an integral part of the mattress construction where the cover of the topper and the mattress are connected to each other. We call this the 'pillow top mattress'. Pillow top mattresses provide an additional upholstery layer sewn into the top of the mattress. This layer can be made of a variety of fiber and foam materials.

A loose topper used as a mini mattress can be handy if you have a mattress that is too hard, and you want to sleep on something that is a bit softer and more comfortable. Also if, for instance, you have lost a lot of weight, your mattress will feel harder and less comfortable: you can then temporarily consider a topper. Furthermore, a topper is useful if you would like a bit more resilience, or want to lie slightly higher in your bed.

In the so-called Scandinavian sleep system, the topper is a necessary component, along with a box spring and the mattress.

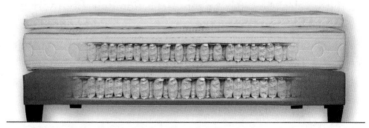

Figure 74 A 'real' Scandinavian sleep system, consisting of a box spring, pocket spring mattress and small mini mattress – the topper.

Slatted bases

Slatted bases are the most popular foundations in Western Europe. They can be installed free-standing on legs, but are usually placed in a bed frame.

A slatted base consists of a wooden or metal frame containing fixed slats or slats that can bounce and sometimes also tilt. The slats are made of wood, fiberglass or a combination of materials and are inserted under pressure into the frame. The number of slats per slatted base can vary substantially: from 14 to more than twice as much. Of course, this also affects the width and the thickness of the slats. Furthermore, curve, resilience or simply color may vary. Sometimes several kinds of slats are placed in a single base: soft slats at the shoulders and adjustable, reinforced slats in the middle area of the body. The slatted base is the support for the mattress and amounts to approximately 60 percent of the total surface area. The remaining 40 percent of open space is necessary for optimal moisture regulation of the mattress. Never lay a mattress on a closed substructure such as a board because this will cause mold formation.

It is impossible to draw conclusions about the quality and reclining comfort of the slatted base, from the number of slats, color, material, thickness, et cetera. But there is a golden rule for conformity: a good slatted base guarantees the highest possible resilience over the entire lying surface. If you lie on the side of your bed, a good slatted base will also guarantee some resilience here.

The slats are mounted on the side in slat suspensions. There are fixed versions, but the better ones are flexible and will also move along when you load the slats.

The more flexible or adjustable the slat suspensions, the more comfortable the sleep system is. Sometimes the slat suspensions can be adjusted to the body shape. Resilient slat suspensions usually increase the comfort when lying on the side of the bed. The hard middle area where two slatted bases are positioned adjacent to each other, will be less perceptible.

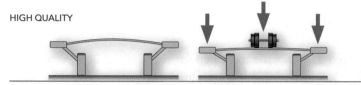

Figure 75.1   The slats and slat suspensions move when loaded.

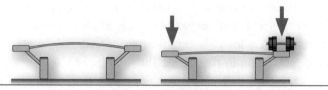

Figure 75.2   The slats and slat suspensions move along when loaded laterally.

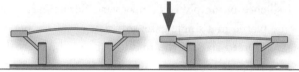

Figure 75.3   Resilient slat suspensions on the side ensure a flexible middle zone when there are two adjacent slatted bases.

LOW QUALITY

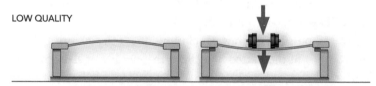

Figure 75.4   The slats and slat suspensions do not move when loaded; only the slat sags.

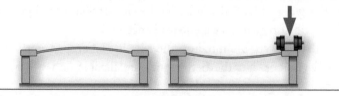

Figure 75.5   The slats and slat suspensions do not move when loaded laterally.

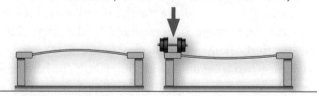

Figure 75.6   Non-resilient slat suspensions on the side have a hard middle zone when there are two adjacent slatted bases.

CHAPTER 6

✗ Tip

In a bed store you can try out the flexibility of the slat suspensions by pushing down on the centre of the slats. A base with slat suspensions that move together with the slats is the best choice. Some higher quality suspensions have adjustable hardness too.

✗ How do you choose a slatted base?

Don't opt for...

- ✗ fixed slats that aren't bouncy.
- ✗ slats that are more than 2.5 inches apart from each other; the support surface for your mattress is then too small.

But do go for...

- ✗ slatted bases which are softer at the level of the shoulders,
- ✗ slatted bases that are reinforced in the middle area,
- ✗ slat suspensions that are flexible or adjustable,
- ✗ slatted bases with maximum resilience over the full surface and also with some resilience at the sides. High quality slatted bed bases are made in Western Europe.

A modern approach to sleep comfort

In this chapter, we will bring together all the topics we have covered so far, and explain how everything you have read in this book fits together. If you are considering buying a new bed, this chapter can serve as a guide. It may also interest you, even if you would just like to check whether your current sleep system suits you.

Scientific research on sleep systems often focuses on the curve of the spinal column: sleep systems that maintain and support the natural curve are satisfactory, others are not. The curve of the spinal column is usually a good indicator to assess the extent to which a sleep system will meet the most important bed parameters. This is undeniably an important factor, but it is certainly not the only one. Based on my own research, expertise and 20 years of experience, I can say that a sleep system must also always be adjusted to a few individual parameters:

× body weight;
× height;
× body mass index or BMI (the ratio between the weight and the square of the height);
× the shoulder, waist and hip widths;
× the mutual relationship between those widths;
× the general body shape;
× the curve of the spinal column.

Based on our current knowledge of sleep comfort, we will now provide a brief overview of the requirements that a good sleep system should meet.

HOW DO I PUT MY SLEEP SYSTEM TOGETHER?

Currently, the most advanced method for putting together a sleep system consists of measuring and analysing the body parameters. The technology is developing rapidly but is still in its infancy – although scientists and the mattress industry have been working hard on it.

But awaiting this technology, you can get a lot of advice in a bed store. The questionnaire below can be used as a guide.

× **Conformity:** Are you a slim person or do you have a larger build? What are the differences between your shoulder, waist and hip widths? What is the shape of your spinal column in front and side view?

× **Firmness:** How tall are you? How much do you weigh? What is your body mass index? Do you have a subjective preference for hard or soft?

× **Moisture regulation:** Do you perspire a lot at night? In other words, what is the difference between your weight before going to bed and upon getting up?

× **Thermal insulation:** Do you prefer to sleep warm or rather cool? Is your bedroom heated? Do you have a cold bedroom or a rather warm one?

× **Health problems:** Do you have health problems that affect your sleep or sleeping position? Do you have neck, back or shoulder pain? Are you allergic to house dust mites?

A good adviser will also take into account your personal preferences. Furthermore, you should always try out the bed extensively. We will now examine in deeper depth each of the criteria we have mentioned above.

SHOULD I SLEEP IN A HARD OR A SOFT BED?

In Chapter 5 we have extensively covered the pros and cons of sleeping on a hard or soft system. Here we will primarily examine how you decide which system will suit you best.

The most important objective criteria to determine the ideal hardness of a sleep system are, as we saw in Chapter 4, body weight and the body mass index. An obese person will obviously sink more deeply into the same mattress than a lean person. The heavier person should therefore opt for a firmer mattress. We have to be careful not to exaggerate: just as extremely soft is not good for sleeping comfort, the same holds for extremely firm.

In the past, when everyone still slept on sagging mattresses and bed bases, hard sleep systems were always advised in cases of chronic lower back pain. More recent studies however, indicate that patients are better served with softer mattresses. These findings are in line with my own experience and research. It is a myth that sleeping on a firm mattress is always the healthiest.

If you nonetheless opt for a harder sleep system, please ensure that this is not contrary to the principle of conformity! A sleep system can be a bit harder as long as it supports the natural position of the spinal column.

The hardness of a sleep system is mainly determined by the mattress, in combination with the bed base. There is a clear interaction between the two. If you combine a soft mattress with a hard bed base, the mattress must be thick enough (guideline value: at least 8 inches) to prevent you from feeling the base and to be able to guarantee basic comfort. The heavier you are, the firmer the mattress will need to be. Thin mattresses have a limited resilience and are best combined with highly conforming bed bases, such as some slatted bases. These bed bases are very popular in Western Europe.

A good mattress should not feel too hard on the hips and shoulders, but it may also not be so soft that a hammock effect is created. If you lie on your side, the mattress should continue to support the waist in such a way that the spinal column forms a straight line.

This can be tried out really well in a bed store. Make sure to wear close-fitting clothes so your body curves can be seen clearly and take someone along who can observe you while you are lying down.

PRESSURE, PRESSURE, PRESSURE!

To explain the interplay of a mattress and a bed base, we have collected a few pressure measurements. The results are significant.

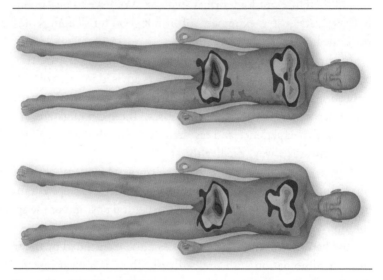

Figures 76 and 77   When taking a pressure measurement on a Bonnell spring mattress in combination with a fixed slatted base, we see extremely high pressure points at the level of the pelvis (above). In the case of a Bonnell spring mattress and a flexible slatted base, the high pressure points are partially offset by the slatted base (below).

Figure 76 represents the pressure on the skin of a test person. The test person is lying on his back on a hard mattress with rigid slats underneath. The pressure zones go from green (light pressure) to yellow and blue to purple (very strong pressure). We see that the highest pressure occurs around the pelvis and the hips. This is because the largest body mass is concentrated there.

In Figure 77, we see the same test person lying on the same mattress, but this time with a flexible slatted base as a support.

In both figures, the pressure at the pelvis is high, but we clearly see that the slatted base has eliminated some of the pressure.

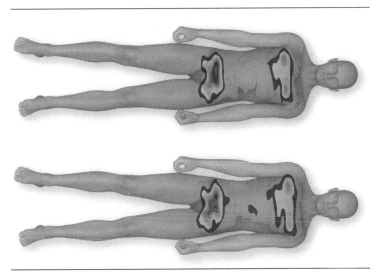

Figures 78 and 79 Above: pressure measurement on a softer mattress in combination with a fixed slatted base, with excessive pressure at the level of the pelvis. Below: pressure measurement on a soft mattress in combination with a flexible slatted base with good pressure distribution.

In Figure 78, a test person is lying supine on a resilient mattress with five comfort zones. The mattress has an elastic cover and is positioned on rigid slats. In Figure 79, we see the test person lying on the same mattress, but this time on a flexible slatted base.

From a comparison between Figures 76 and 78, we can deduce that the resilient mattress does the better job: there are fewer zones of high pressure in Figure 78, while the foundation in both systems consists of the same base of rigid slats. However, the pressure at the level of the pelvis is still too high with the resilient mattress. Pressure measurement 79 shows a good pressure distribution: the best mattress in this experiment, combined with a flexible slatted base.

A small warning: pressure measurements provide an indication of the hardness. Pressure mats belong in laboratories and not in showrooms! However, they don't tell us whether the spinal column is supported in such a way that it can maintain its natural shape. For that we must look at our next factor: conformity.

HOW DO I MAKE SURE MY BODY IS WELL SUPPORTED?

The extent to which your sleep system adapts to your body shape is what we call conformity (Figure 80). All sleep systems must have a high conformity, but how they achieve that depends on your body shape, the weight distribution of your body and the shape of your spinal column as seen from the front and from the side.

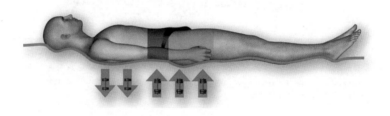

Figure 80   Highly conforming sleep systems give more support at the level of the heaviest body zones and are also softer at the level of the shoulders.

Let's just illustrate this by means of two test persons with very different body shapes.

A slim woman

Our first subject is a slim woman with broad shoulders and hips and a narrow waist. She has a hollow lower back.

CHAPTER 7

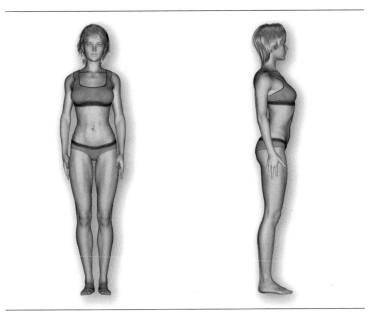

Figure 81 A slim woman with a hollow back.

The narrower the waist relative to the hips and shoulders, the higher the conformity of the sleep combination, in particular of the mattress, must be (Figure 82).

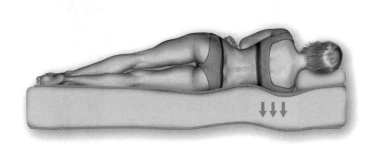

Figure 82 Soft shoulder zones in the sleep system increase the conformity in the case of this woman.

If you look at our test person lying on her side, you understand immediately why: her shoulders and hips stick out relative to the body plane and her waist deviates inwards. Shoulders and hips must therefore be able to sink sufficiently into the sleep system. At the same time the waist must be supported to prevent the spinal column from sagging. Viewed from the back, it could never form a straight line – which is its natural shape, after all. The shoulder zone of the mattress will usually be the softest.

An obese man

Our second subject is a small, obese man without pronounced body contours. The curves of his vertebral column are flattened (see Figure 83).

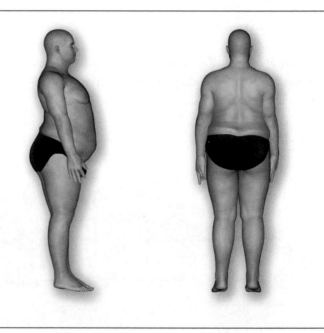

Figure 83 A small, obese man without pronounced body contours.

CHAPTER 7

The conformity requirements for this man's sleep system will be lower. The difference in width between hips, shoulders and waist is considerably less so the mattress and the bed base need to adapt less. The sleep system will need to be somewhat more sturdy and harder because the man has a higher body mass index.

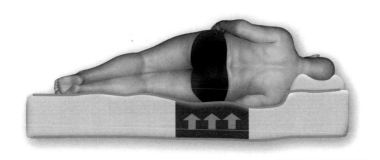

Figure 84   Reinforced middle zones increase the conformity in the case of this man.

People with a heavy hip and pelvic region might best opt for a mattress with a reinforced middle zone (see Figure 84) – they may even consider choosing a bed base with an adapted construction.

It is also important that the sleep system attempts to maintain the man's flattened vertebral column curves. A sleep system should not attempt to correct, instead it should adapt precisely to the unique body shape of the sleeper.

THREE ZONES

A sleep system with good conformity has three hardness zones: at the level of the shoulders, at the waist and at the hips. An excellent combination for this obese man is: soft at the shoulders and hard at the waist and the hips. Obese people do not have any hips that protrude from the body plane so the mattress does not need a soft hip zone to allow them to sink into (see Figure 85). The two hard zones serve to compensate for the weight of the man. If those zones were too soft, the man would sink into the bed, and come to lie in a dip.

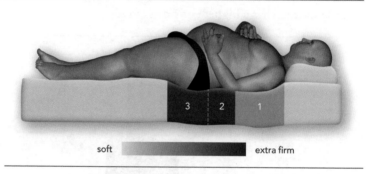

soft ▬▬▬▬▬▬▬▬▬▬ extra firm

Figure 85   Increased conformity with reinforced middle zones 2 and 3 and flexible shoulder zone 1.

The best option for our slim woman would be to choose this combination: soft shoulder zone, hard waist and soft hips. Her shoulders and hips, which protrude from her body plane, can now sink sufficiently into the soft zones of the mattress, while the curve of her waist is supported by the harder zone. The hip zone can be softened, for instance, by more yielding of the slatted base in that location (see Figure 86). In any event, you usually get the highest conformity in sleep systems with soft shoulder zones.

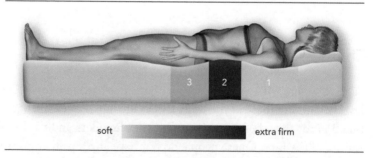

soft ▬▬▬▬▬▬▬▬▬▬ extra firm

Figure 86   Increased conformity with reinforced lumbar zone 2 and softer zones 1 and 3.

According to the European Consumer Organisations, 60 to 80 percent of conformity is determined by the mattress, the remaining 20 to 40 percent by the bed base. Some manufacturers assert, on the other hand, that this is fifty-fifty. Whatever is correct: the overall conformity of your sleep system is determined by mattress, bed base and pillow (in Chapter 9 we will deal extensively with the pillow). The bed base must flexibly adapt to your body shape and to changes in position. The general rule is: the thinner the mattress, the more important the conformity of the bed base.

In recent years, sleep systems are becoming increasingly adaptable to the individual in question. The advantage of this adaptability is that you can really create a customised sleep system and that you can adjust it afterwards if, for instance, you have gained a few pounds. Some manufacturers make so-called 'self-regulating' bed bases; they are said to automatically adjust to your sleeping positions. Note: check carefully to what extent they are softer at the shoulders and firmer at the level of the lower back. To what extent they are better we do not know yet. The research about this is still in development.

HOW DO I ENSURE GOOD MOISTURE REGULATION?

If you perspire at night, it is best to sleep on a bed with good moisture regulation. That means that it readily absorbs moisture, stores it and then releases it again to the environment. If those conditions are met the bed will never feel moist or damp.

Every sleep system has two major moisture buffers. The bed linen and the outer textile layers of the mattress form the first line of defense for a good moisture regulation. Anyone who sweats a lot, for instance, will be best off opting for a mattress with thick, airy and/or absorbing top layers. The moisture is then quickly removed and the contact between the mattress and skin will remain comfortably dry. Regarding the bed linen, duvets filled with duck or goose down are a good choice. It's also advisable to use mattress protectors, fitted sheets and duvet covers made of 100 percent cotton.

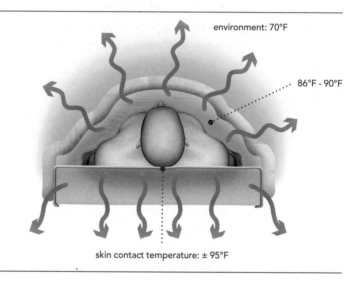

environment: 70°F

86°F - 90°F

skin contact temperature: ± 95°F

Figure 87 The bed linen and the mattress have a big influence on the moisture and heat regulation around the body.

The second moisture buffer is the inner structure of the mattress. The goal here is also absorbing moisture, storing and then releasing it to the environment (see Figure 87). Innerspring mattresses, because of the interior open construction provide generally a better moisture buffer than foam mattresses, which consist of one large block of foam. Much depends on the quality of the foam used.

Anyway, it is advisable to give your mattress the chance to get rid of the nightly build-up of moisture during the day. You can do this by leaving your bed uncovered not making your bed untill bedtime. Warm air can absorb more water vapor than cold air, so you can safely leave the heat on.

Of course you also have to air the bedroom occasionally in order to get rid of that moist air again. In homes that are very well insulated you may need active ventilation for this.

Slatted bed bases probably allow for better ventilation than box springs.

HOW DO I ENSURE GOOD BED TEMPERATURE?

People who easily feel cold or who sleep in an unheated room need a sleep system with good thermal insulation, otherwise their bodies cool down too much.

Of course, duvets and blankets play an important role here, but we should certainly not forget the mattress. High resilience foam and latex mattresses have a high insulation value. Innerspring mattress score slightly weaker than the rest, but on the flip side, this means that they are a good choice for people who easily feel too warm at night.

The materials which have been incorporated into the mattress cover also play a role. Wool, for instance, is a good thermal insulator because of its frizzy structure.

ALLERGIC TO HOUSE DUST MITES?

Anyone who is allergic to house dust mites or suffers from asthma would be best off choosing a cover that is filled with materials, that is removable and can be washed at 140°F. Some covers also constitute a barrier for the mites. More explanation about that in Chapter 10.

JUST COMBINE IT!

So for good sleeping comfort, you need a good mattress and a good bed base, but the two must also be fine-tuned to each other. Basically, it is possible to combine any bed base – except for a few types of slatted bases – with a suitable type of mattress.

Slatted bases

» Innerspring mattresses

The larger the support surface of the bed base, the more you will benefit from the properties of the innerspring mattress. A slatted base combined with such a mattress must thus have sufficient slats (28 or more). Furthermore, the distance between the slats must be kept as small as possible (maximum 2 to 2.5 inches). Flat slatted bases can be combined with all kinds of innerspring mattresses, but on an electrically adjustable base, you are best off using the very flexible pocket spring mattresses with stretch covers – stretch covers around mattresses increase the reclining comfort and the flexibility.

Pocket spring mattresses with ergonomic zones increase the conformity of the system.

» Foam and latex mattresses

Flexible slatted bases conform very well. You can use them with all types of mattresses, but they are best combined with foam and latex mattresses. Those have a higher flexibility, so you get a more comfortable result from your slatted base.

It is better not to combine an adjustable slatted base with a polyether mattress because those are firmer than High Resilience foam (HR) and latex mattresses: you then cancel out the action of the flexible slats.

Latex and HR foam mattresses with ergonomic zones – for instance, a soft shoulder zone and a firm hip zone – increase the conformity of the whole system.

Box springs

Box springs are usually less conforming than a good slatted bed base. It is best to combine them with a sufficiently thick mattress – at least 8 inches is the rule of thumb. Box springs are less permeable to moisture than slatted bases. Pocket spring mattresses – which absorb moisture exceedingly well and release it again to the air – are thus the most suitable here. You may also lay HR foam and latex mattresses on box springs, again assuming that they are sufficiently thick, because most box springs do not score too well on conformity. To compensate for the less efficient moisture regulation of the box spring, it is advisable to use very good bed linen and a mattress cover that is quilted with moisture-regulating filling. Ventilating the room very well will be an ongoing task for box spring sleepers.

IN SUMMARY: COMBINATION TIPS

Slatted bases

× Can be combined with all mattress types assuming that the support surface is sufficiently large.
× Conformity from moderate to high is possible.

Box spring and divan

× Can be combined with all mattress types.
× Moderate conformity.
× To date, there is a limited range of box springs with good conformity available in stores. You can compensate for this with a sufficiently thick, highly conforming mattress.

Adjustable bed base

× Should not be combined with Bonnell spring mattresses.
× Preferably should be combined with foam, latex or pocket spring mattresses, finished with elastic covers.

CHAPTER 8

Neck pain and the pillow

Neck pain is a common complaint. About 30 percent of people suffer from it sometimes – women more than men – and there is also a peak between the ages of 50 and 60. Just as with back pain we often find no direct cause. The cause might be a muscle strain due to an unexpected movement or facet pain due to prolonged poor posture at work or during sleep. The cause is difficult to determine because scientists have described more than 50 causes! Often neck pain is accompanied by reduced sleep quality, muscle stiffness and pain radiating to the head, arm or shoulders.

Many neck complaints are due to an incorrect sleeping position which puts the joint capsules and ligaments of the cervical vertebrae under tension for a long time. An unsuitable pillow or mattress can aggravate things even more. Time to look at the problem more thoroughly.

THE CERVICAL SPINE

The cervical spine consists of seven vertebrae and forms the connection between the skull and the trunk. It is much more mobile than the rest of the spinal column because it needs to facilitate the head movements. These vertebrae are somewhat smaller than those in the rest of the spinal column, but here too, the inter-vertebral discs will have to absorb a lot of pressure due to the relatively high weight of the head, approximately 13 lbs. Of all inter-vertebral disc disorders, about 36 percent occur in the cervical spine. We find the majority in the lowest cervical vertebrae, probably because they are most often involved in movement. The lowest cervical vertebrae form the transition to the relatively rigid thoracic spine, which results in some additional strain.

Another striking difference of the cervical vertebrae with respect to the lower back: the transverse protrusions at the side of the cervical vertebrae have holes. These holes form a tunnel through which the blood vessels run to and from our head.

Shoulders and neck area

Humans have a fairly unique neck and shoulder anatomy – which evolved when our ancestors started walking upright. In quadrupeds, the shoulders are mainly held in place by muscles. But when you walk on two feet, this no longer suffices: you need stronger structures to withstand gravity. That's why, to begin with, we developed a broad and fairly flat rib cage. In most animals (picture the skeleton of a dog) the rib cage is deep and narrow. Furthermore, our clavicles have become long and sturdy: they connect the sternum to the shoulder and offer permanent support to the shoulders (see Figure 88). The clavicles are usually very small or even absent in other animals. Together with the shoulder blades, the clavicles also ensure that we can do something very unique: we can fully rotate our arms. As a result, we can execute movements that are impossible for most other animals, for example throwing, climbing with our arms or swimming on our backs. Being able to execute those movements has consequences for sleep, and strain can lead to neck and shoulder problems.

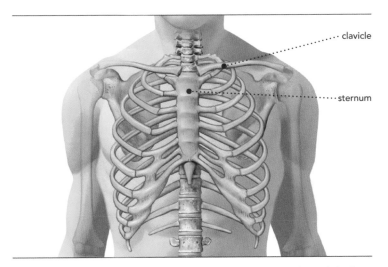

labels: clavicle, sternum

Figure 88 The long and strong clavicles serve as a lever, so that, together with the flat, wide rib cage, they position the shoulders high and sideways.

Brachial plexus

In the neck and shoulder area there is yet another important structure: the *plexus brachialis* or brachial plexus, a network of nerves and blood vessels serving the shoulders and arms.

From the fourth cervical vertebra to the first thoracic vertebra, the nerves emerge from the spinal cord and braid themselves together into the brachial plexus. The brachial plexus then passes first in between some muscles and then dives into the narrow space between the clavicle and the upper rib towards the arm (see Figure 89). During sleep, strands of the brachial plexus may become stretched and come under pressure due to uncomfortable positions, too hard a bed or an unsuitable pillow. With increased muscle tension, the openings through which the plexus runs may become even smaller, causing pressure on the nerves. Fortunately, symptoms arising in this way can generally be quickly resolved. And this kind of pain usually disappears when you get up – because the load on the structures disappears.

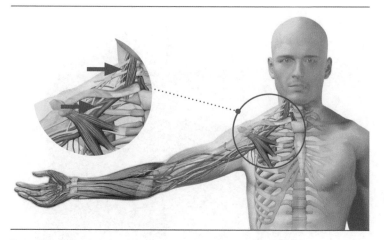

Figure 89   The brachial plexus, the sensitive network of nerves and blood vessels, starts from the cervical vertebrae and then runs between the muscles and under the clavicle to the arm.

× TOS

Compression of the plexus is called thoracic outlet syndrome (TOS) – there are even outpatient clinics that treat only plexus injuries! The thoracic outlet is the outlet from the thorax (the medical name for chest) to the arm. You will probably recognize the symptoms immediately: a tingling or sleeping sensation in the fingers, hand and/ or arm on one side of your body. Note! These symptoms may also occur if there is pressure on the nerve roots at the level of the cervical vertebrae.

The cervical spine during sleep

Because of the very specific construction of the cervical vertebrae, the shoulders and the structures around, is it important that we adequately support the cervical spine and the head during sleep. The entire sleep system is responsible for that, with the pillow as the final piece to consider.

How it should not be

Neck pain can occur because you are lying on an unadjusted or unsuitable sleep system or when sleeping in a position that puts strain on the neck. We will give a few examples of common cases.

It will be difficult to find adequate support for the neck when sleeping on a surface that is too hard. Moreover, the underlying shoulder will shift in the direction of the head, up to the chin or even higher (Figure 90). Because of its great width combined with its lower weight, the shoulder girdle fails to sink sufficiently deep into the mattress. As a result, it will push the pillow away. The lowest cervical vertebrae are then insufficiently supported and will bend, causing the spinal column structures to come under pressure.

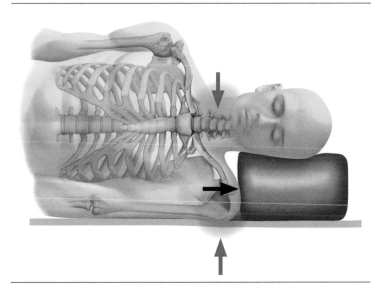

Figure 90   On a bed which is too hard, the shoulder shifts upwards, causing the cervical vertebrae to be insufficiently supported. This can lead to pain.

Poor lying positions, such as the 'hurray position' (both arms above the head) can also cause too much pressure on the brachial plexus.

As a result, you can feel tingling and pain in the fingers – this will usually wake you up. The tingling will usually disappear when you change position. The ligaments around your shoulder joints can also get subjected to excessive pressure and tension.

When lying on your stomach you will have to turn your head sideways, therefore turning your cervical vertebrae. That rotation, combined with hyperextension of the vertebrae, can put tension on the nerve roots (Figure 91). When lying on your stomach, it is preferable to use no pillow at all or just a thin one.

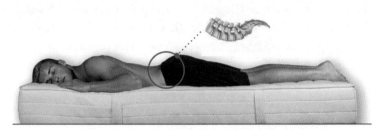

Figure 91 Lying on your stomach, the lumbar curvature is usually greater and the cervical vertebrae come under stress.

Lying on your back with your head on a pillow that is too thick might lead to tension (Figure 92) and strain on the soft tissue. Overloading the structures in the neck can also cause shoulder problems.

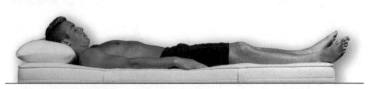

Figure 92 The use of a pillow that is too thick results in a bending load on the cervical vertebrae.

The damage

A well-known example of neck pain is the spontaneous acute twisted neck or *torticollis*: soft tissue will be overloaded, resulting in a painful swelling. The body reacts to this by locally increasing the muscle tension, and thus creating a natural brace around the injury. The head is slanted and can, because of this blocking, no longer move. Torticollis is very painful and often occurs in children between the ages of five and fourteen.

Sometimes local neck pain or tension evolves into a diffuse pain difficult to pinpoint. It is also often accompanied by shoulder pain and pain radiating to the head or the arm.

Characteristic for neck symptoms is that they often worsen at night. The pain can occur both at night and in the morning and can lead to sleep disorders. As a result you will not be well rested. Lack of sleep might increase the pain and therefore your sleep will be even worse. This is a vicious circle. Localised small lesions can spread and thus become chronic.

My own research shows that optimalisation of the sleep system – with special attention to the combination of mattress and pillow – makes an important contribution to the recovery from sleep-related shoulder and neck symptoms.

THE PILLOW

The sleep system consists of the mattress, the bed base and the pillow. And just like with the mattress and the bed base, the pillow must also meet certain conditions.

Conformity and hardness

To begin with, the pillow needs to support both the neck and head continuously. When lying on your side, the lowest cervical vertebrae should form a straight line with the rest of the spinal column. This way, the neck is the least strained. When lying on your back, the pillow should retain the forward curve of the cervical vertebrae (see Figure 95).

During the deep sleep phase, when muscle relaxation is maximal, the natural position of the cervical vertebrae must be supported as fully as possible – the muscles are then no longer able to do their normal work.

If, by lying on your back; you only support the neck and not the head, the natural curve of the cervical vertebrae will become much more pronounced. This is called hyperextension, and it can lead to joint pain (Figure 93). So always use a pillow that supports both the neck and head.

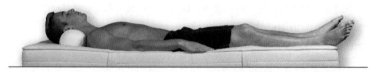

Figure 93 When only the neck zone is supported, this often gives rise to a stretching load.

The pillow must be highly conforming and fill the hollow space of the body between the shoulder girdle and the head so that the head can rest in a saucer-shaped dimple. The aim for good support is located at the base of the neck, just above the clavicle, at the level of the lower three cervical vertebrae (Figure 94).

To determine the conformity of the pillow, the construction of the shoulder girdle, the shape of the cervical vertebrae and the comfort characteristics of the mattress and bed base are taken into account.

The hardness of the pillow yet again depends on the weight of your head.

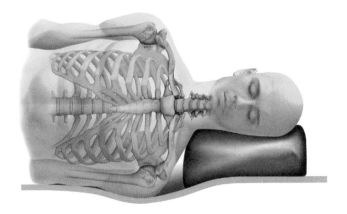

Figure 94   By lying on a highly conforming sleep system with a soft shoulder zone, the pillow can support the cervical vertebrae.

✗ Tip

Ideally, you should try out your pillow on a mattress such as the one you have at home. Try it out when lying on your back and on your side, and check whether when lying on your side, your cervical vertebrae form a straight line with the rest of your spinal column. You will soon notice that this is only possible if your bed is soft enough at the level of the shoulders.

Moisture regulation

The same requirements apply to the pillow as to the mattress and the bed base. The moisture that we evaporate must be absorbed and dissipated, so that we do not end up lying on a damp underlayer.

Naturally, the cover of the pillow plays a role in this, but the filling is the most important. Down pillows, for instance, transport water vapor better than pillows that are filled with standard polyurethane foam or latex.

Heat regulation

The thermal insulation capacity is also strongly depending on the filling. Pillows with stronger thermal insulation will lead more readily to a disturbed sleep than cooler pillows. According to Japanese researchers, cooler pillows lower your body temperature, because they allow your head to feel less warm. This will result in deeper sleep. For the time being, however, there isn't much comparable research material available. If you are in doubt about what to buy, ask if you can take home some pillows to try out, or request an exchange guarantee.

Types of pillows

There is an abundant range of pillows on the market. What type of pillow will suit you best depends, among other things, on your cervical spine, your sleep habits, your body weight, your shoulder width, the length of your neck and the elasticity of the mattress/bed base combination at the level of your shoulders. How high and firm a good pillow should be cannot be captured in a general rule.

If you lie on your back, the pillow must accommodate the differences in height between the posterior part of the skull, the deepest point of the cervical vertebral column and the bulging of the thoracic vertebral column (Figure 95). If you lie on your side, the pillow must accommodate the differences in height between the ear and the shoulder neckline. How far the shoulders sink into the mattress is highly dependent on the hardness of the shoulder zone of the mattress and the type of bed base. The highest point of the pillow is situated under the neck, the lowest under the head.

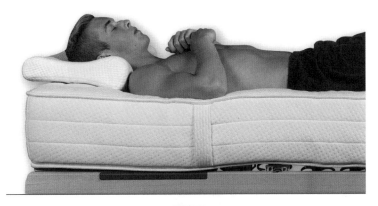

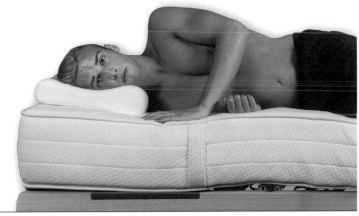

Figure 95 Best choose a pillow according to your own body structure and the hardness of the sleep system at the level of the shoulder zone.

» Dimensions

In the US, pillows are common in these three sizes: Standard (20 x 26 inches), Queen (20 x 30 inches), and King (20 x 36 inches). In the US, a less common size is Jumbo or Full (20 x 28 inches), which is larger than the Standard size but smaller than the Queen size and the Euro (26 x 26 inches). Common pillow size in the UK is 20 x 30 inches.

» Materials

Good quality pillows have a cotton cover with different types of natural and/or synthetic filling: polyester, HR foam, latex, down, wool, cotton, feathers etc.

Pillows can also be filled with air and water or small pocket springs, but unfortunately discussing all this will require much more space.

✗ Synthetic fillings

The most commonly used synthetic fillings are polyester and ball-shaped polyester fibers (Figure 96). Ball-shaped polyester fibers will increase the resilience, feel like down and do not tangle easily after washing. They can be washed at 140°F.

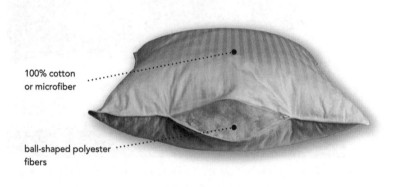

100% cotton
or microfiber

ball-shaped polyester
fibers

Figure 96   Pillow filled with hypoallergenic ball-shaped polyester fibers.

✗ Natural fillings

Pillows are often filled with natural materials such as down and feathers (Figure 97).

Down and feather pillows are easy to shake up so you can adjust the shape of the pillow to your body shape and your preferences.

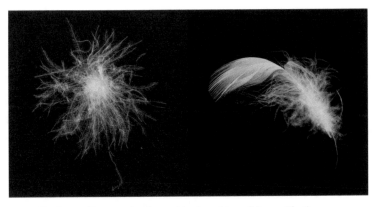

Figure 97   Down pillows consist of a combination of down flakes and feathers.

✗ Foam and latex fillings

Just like with mattresses, the choice exist between synthetic or natural latex fillings, or a blend of the two. Latex pillows usually have good conformity and pressure distribution and good thermal insulation properties. They are available in all shapes, hardnesses and thicknesses.

In recent years, HR foam pillows that score as well as the best latex pillows are available.

The best types of memory foam pillows (the material that yields under the influence of pressure and temperature) score well on heat and moisture regulation, but whether they adequately support the head and neck remains questionable for the time being. The shape of the pillows will play an important role here. You should certainly ask for an exchange guarantee if you are contemplating to buy a memory foam pillow.

THE ORTHOPAEDIC PILLOW

If traditional pillows do not support your neck sufficiently, you might consider an orthopaedic pillow. This ensures correct support for the cervical vertebrae and head. The neck zone is usually sturdier than the head zone. They come in different shapes, materials, thickness and hardness and often have built-in neck support systems. In case of some orthopaedic pillows, the neck section is actually higher than the centrally positioned head section.

My own research shows that orthopaedic pillows, whether or not combined with mattresses equipped with soft shoulder zones, lead to a decrease in neck and shoulder complaints and make a positive contribution to the quality of sleep. Many people have to get used to their unusual shape. That may take a few days to a few weeks.

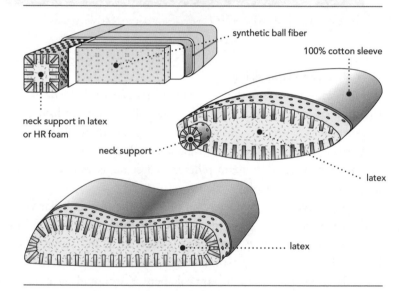

Figure 98 Some examples of orthopaedic pillows: a pillow divided into compartments with integrated neck support in HR foam or high-quality latex (top), a latex pillow with built-in neck support (middle) and a molded orthopaedic pillow in natural latex (bottom).

CHAPTER 9

Sleeping and resting positions

So far we have mainly discussed sleep systems, but naturally your lying and sleeping position also plays a role in the development and continuation of back pain and sleep problems. We will look at that further on in this chapter.

A good sleeping and lying position is important to our physical and mental wellbeing. There are no rules for an 'ideal' sleeping position: that differs from person to person, and what's more, we often unconsciously change positions during our sleep.

We all seem to have a favorite position for falling asleep, a position in which we feel comfortable and relaxed. People with back pain will seek a position for falling asleep in which they feel the least pain. The fetal position, lying on one's side (Figure 99), is often recommended, because you are lying in a very stable way. Go lie on your side and pull your legs up until there is a 135 degree angle between the thighbone and the trunk. With a 90 degree angle at the knees, you get the best muscle relaxation of the hip flexors and extensors. According to researchers, that is the normal position for the lower part of the spinal column in a weightless state. The hands may optionally be placed between the legs.

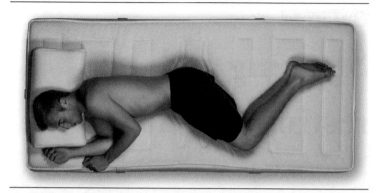

Figure 99 The fetal position lying on one's side with slightly raised hips and knees and head support is a good position for falling asleep.

Once we have fallen asleep, the so-called sleep motor skills come into play: we change position regularly, without complete muscle relaxation ever taking place. In eight hours time, we change position twenty to forty times. The movements vary from a simple repositioning of the arm to changing sides. The number of changes in position varies greatly from person to person. What is a normal amount of changes of position for one person can be more or less for another. In recent years, there has been more research into the relationship between changes in position and sleep quality. This research has shown that the sleep motor skills are linked in one way or another to REM sleep: the big changes in position take place before and after REM sleep.

THE FAVORITE POSITIONS

About 65 percent of all people sleep lying on their sides and lying half the time on their sides and half the time on their stomach. Approximately 30 percent prefer lying on their back and 5 percent on their stomach. These preferences may change with age. Lying on one's stomach – a position that is not recommended – for instance, decreases with age; lying on one's side increases. Lying on one's back remains relatively constant. Of those people who prefer lying on their side, most lie on their right side. That proportion also increases with age. Older people generally change position less frequently and also sleep less.

ACCEPTABLE LYING POSITIONS

We continue with an overview of acceptable lying and sleeping positions for people with or without back pain.

Prone position (lying on your stomach)

Sleeping in prone position or on the stomach is the worst possible position for the cervical spine. For most people, the natural curve of the lumbar vertebrae will become stronger in that position, so that the pressure on the facet joints increases – gravity and extended legs encourage this effect. As a result, especially in the morning hours, lower back pain may occur. Belly sleepers lying on soft mattresses are often confronted with this.

Furthermore, lying prone causes increased pressure on the intestines and lungs. The contents of the abdomen push against the diaphragm, which can even lead to breathing difficulties.

If you lie on your stomach, you need to turn your head sideways, otherwise your mouth and nose are covered and you cannot breathe. The cervical spine is therefore required to twist as far as it can. This puts pressure on the facet joints at the rear of the upper cervical vertebrae and the ligaments are stretched forcefully.

Blood vessels that supply blood to the head and the brain run left and right of the cervical vertebrae. If there is extreme torsion on the cervical vertebrae, these blood vessels may come under too much pressure, which can lead to headache, dizziness and other symptoms.

Conclusion: you would do well to avoid sleeping on your stomach. The strain on the soft tissues and the facet joints of cervical vertebrae and lumbar vertebrae leads to morning stiffness. And if you pull your arms up too high, while lying on your belly, overloading may also occur at the level of the shoulders, also with possible pain symtoms.

Consequently, other joint and muscle tension may also happen around your shoulders and neck, and breathing difficulties may occur. Some researchers even suggest that lying on your stomach is often the cause of increased back pain.

Yet some people experience subjective feelings of comfort when lying on their belly. Often they embrace their pillow. If a person feels reduced pain only in this belly position, it goes without saying that he must adopt that position.

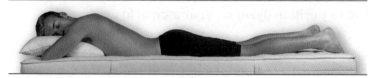

Figure 100 Embracing the pillow lying on your belly gives a pleasant feeling of comfort, but overloads the lower back.

» Comfortable positions

Anyone who has neck and back pain should try to avoid sleeping on the stomach. If you are nonetheless unable to unlearn it, there are a few tips to somewhat reduce the pressure on neck and back.

× Try sleeping without a pillow or with a very thin pillow.

× Place a pillow under the lower abdomen and pelvis (see Figure 101). This is a simple way to flatten the lower back. Sometimes this position is recommended in acute lower back pain, although it does increase the pressure on the abdomen.

× The curvature of the lumbar vertebrae flattens out if you draw up your knee and hip to the side your head is facing. You can also raise your arm and omit the pillow so that the curve of the neck flattens out (Figure 102). If you now place another pillow under your abdomen, you are lying in a more stable position – the so-called half prone or half lateral position (see Figure 103). Whether or not it is better to use a pillow in this position is something you best try out for yourself. People unconsciously assume different positions and experiment with pillows in order to exert as little strain as possible on the spinal column.

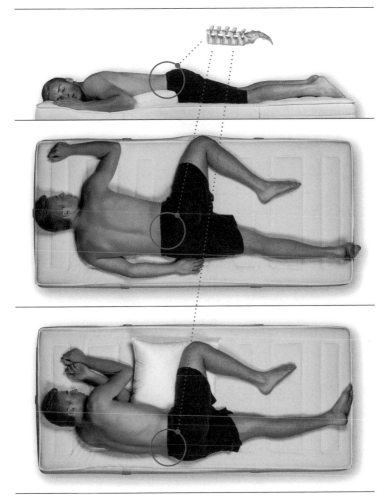

Figures 101, 102 and 103   A number of different lying positions with flattening of the lower back.

There are also large pillows available that fully support the trunk: they are called boomerang pillows; in the UK, usually V-shaped pillows. They replace the pillows we were just talking about. They are also frequently used by pregnant women during sleep (see Figure 104).

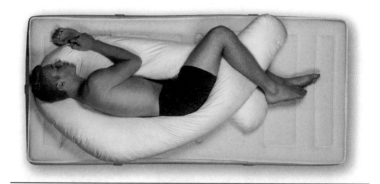

Figure 104　The V-shaped pillow guarantees a stable, comfortable lying position.

Lateral position (lying on your side)

Lying on your side is the most common sleeping position. If the spinal column is supported correctly, it is also a great position for your back - the entire sleep system does have to have a high conformity.

» Left or right?

The lateral position has the advantage that no invasive pressure on blood vessels or intestines arises. When lying on the left side, the weight of the liver, which is situated on the right, does press on the stomach and lungs, but that does not have any major consequences. If you don't have any back pain symptoms, it doesn't matter whether you sleep on your left or on your right side.

» Not twisting

Compared to lying on your back, the lateral position is less stable: the center of gravity of your body is higher and the support surface smaller. However, arms and legs can act as stabilisers and increase the support surface. The pelvis and the shoulder girdle may safely rotate slightly about the longitudinal axis so they end up lying more in a half lateral position – but both in the same direction and to the same extent.

In any case, avoid a lateral lying position in which the spinal column is twisted (Figure 105). This happens especially if you lie in a lateral position with your lower arm behind your back – a position that should absolutely be avoided. Your trunk is twisted forward, with the result that both your shoulders end up lying flat on the bed. That leads to a big rotational strain on several thoracic and cervical vertebrae. You can compare it with wringing out a cloth: you squeeze the fluid from the inter-vertebral discs and the ligaments come under increased pressure. This position also often gives rise to arm and shoulder aches.

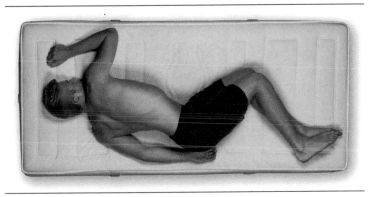

Figure 105   Poor lateral lying positions, in which the spinal column is twisted, often give rise to back symptoms.

» Comfortable positions

Below are a few side-lying positions that are good for the back and are perceived as very relaxed and pleasant.

×   When lying on your side, your upper leg sometimes has the tendency to slide down. Your pelvis then twists along with it, which is not a good thing. In order to avoid that, it's best to place a pillow between the knees. This way, you also avoid undesirable tension in the pelvic muscles (Figure 106). If you now pull up your knees towards your trunk, the angle at the level of the hip joint decreases and flattens the curvature of the lumbar vertebrae (Figure 107). Many patients with lower back pain may experience this as a very relaxing position. Medical practitioners recommend this position for patients whose back pain decreases when they bend forwards while standing - for instance, in the case of facet pain symptoms. For some people, this position does cause tension around the joint between the sacrum and the hips if the upper legs are pulled up too far. You can easily try out for yourself how high you need to pull up your legs to achieve a comfortable position.

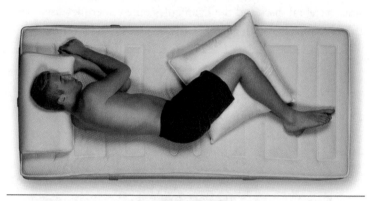

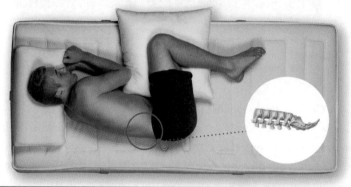

Figures 106 and 107 Comfortable side-lying positions by placing a pillow to counteract twisting at lower back level.

× Anyone who has back pain on one side will sleep best on the non-painful side while pulling up the upper leg. To prevent twisting of the spinal column and of the connections between the spinal column and the pelvis, place a pillow under the top leg (Figure 108).

If you do not like a pillow under your leg but still want to achieve a stable sleeping position, you would do better lying in half lateral position or half prone position. Then pull up the top leg, and if desired, you can put a pillow under your abdomen (Figure 109).

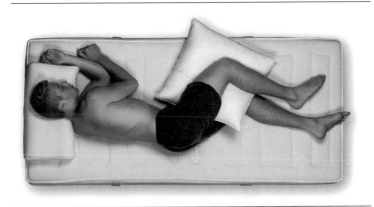

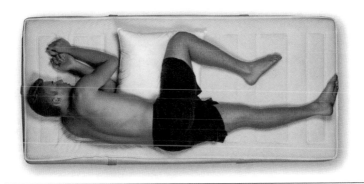

Figures 108 and 109   Comfortable side-lying positions by placing a pillow to counteract twisting at lower back level.

×   Yet another possibility is to sleep on the non-painful side of the back and pull up the leg lying below. The thigh of the top leg will then end up lying over the middle of the thigh and calf of the bottom leg. This leads to a comfortable sleeping position, which will reduce the load on the facet joints throughout the night (Figure 110).

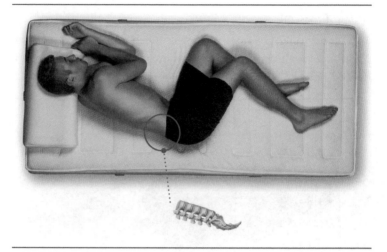

Figure 110 Sleeping position in which mainly the bottom leg is pulled up.

The three positions that we have just described are often recommended to people who have undergone a hernia surgery.

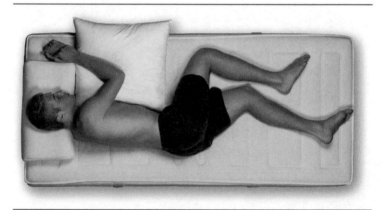

Figure 111 Stable side-lying position with a pillow between the arms to counteract sideways twisting movements.

× Patients with problems at the height of the shoulder sleep best on the pain-free shoulder, possibly with a pillow under the upper elbow and forearm (Figure 111).

Supine position (lying on your back)

The supine position is the most stable position. It also distributes the body weight over the largest possible surface, allowing the muscles maximal relaxation. Anyone who sleeps in a supine position would do well to support his neck and head with a pillow.

When lying supine, the intestines may possibly exert slight pressure on underlying blood vessels and organs. Snoring also occurs much more often in the supine position: gravity presses the tongue and the lower jaw downwards, making it more difficult to breath.

If a patient can only lie on his back and is in pain, he may attempt to fall asleep by making use of a positioning pillow. When one or two pillows are placed under the knee, the lumbar curve is more flattenend (Figure 112). If the pain gets worse when bending forward while standing, a position with a normal or increased lumbar curvature is recommended.

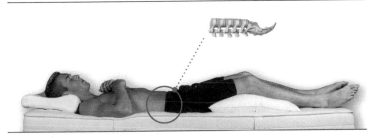

Figure 112   By placing one or more pillows under the hollow of the knee, the lumbar curvature flattens more.

Sleeping with your arms behind your head or with your head resting on your arms is not a good idea. That position leads to an excessive lumbar curvature and could cause arm and shoulder complaints (Figure 113). It further could disrupt the blood circulation in some tendons and could overload the shoulder joints – even to the point where tingling, numbness and a burning sensation might occur. If you already have painful shoulders or arms, you should definitely avoid this position.

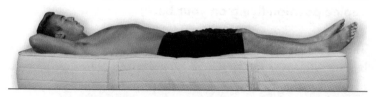

Figure 113   Uncomfortable position with overloading of the shoulder joint and lower back.

BED REST FOR LOWER BACK PAIN

In the remainder of this chapter, we will talk about lower back pain and bed rest, a controversial subject about which the last word has not been said.

Formerly, staying in bed was a medical imperative for patients with lower back pain. In the early 1980's, doubt arose about the therapeutic usefulness of staying in bed. However, undeniable physical changes take place with bed rest which could accelerate the recovery.

Bed rest reduces the pressure in the inter-vertebral discs and the pressure and tensile forces on the ligaments and muscles which surround the spinal column. When we are lying down, our weight is also distributed over a much larger area than when we stand or sit, consequently excessive heavy strain on superficial blood vessels, muscles, joints and bone parts can be avoided.

From a therapeutic point of view, it is therefore important that people with lower back pain can often take on a good sleeping position. A lot of positions that we have discussed above are part of that.

But if the bed rest will go on for too long, there will be consequences that are often more difficult to combat than the original ailment: your bones will weaken, your muscles will slacken and your condition will deteriorate. This can significantly complicate the rehabilitation. In addition, your joints will get stiffer after one or two weeks of bed rest. Elderly and obese people will also be at risk of circulatory disorders.

How long should a patient stay in bed?

Patients with back pain resulting from their daily activities are usually advised to rest for at least twenty minutes each day. The best time for this is after lunch. Anyone who has serious back pain should rest a few times a day.

Sometimes the back pain is so severe that you are unable to do anything else than staying in bed, for instance, if there is an acute and severe nerve root disorder with pain radiating to the legs – such patients feel pain at the slightest movement. Lying alleviates their suffering because the pressure in the inter-vertebral disc decreases, the size of the inter-vertebral space increases and the nerve root is therefore less irritated. That gives the body the opportunity to fight inflammation and to start the healing process. Nevertheless, even in such case, a patient should stay in bed no longer than two to three days. This way the recovery will be faster than with longer periods of bed rest. The message remains: the less, the better, even with acute nerve root complaints!

The most recent studies, however, indicate that even such short periods of bed rest do not always guarantee a faster recovery. Comparative research among patients with acute back pain who either remained active or stayed in bed has demonstrated that the active group went back to work faster, felt less pain and functioned better than the bed rest group.

Another study showed that after one hour of bed rest the inter-vertebral disc had already been rehydrated by nearly 50 percent. You only get 100 percent rehydration in asymptomatic patients after four days of bed rest!

If they had not stayed in bed, they would probably have reached the 100 percent mark considerably earlier because body movements promote rehydration. For chronic back pain sufferers, bed rest as therapy is also inadvisable because it causes loss of muscle mass and your condition will deteriorate. Here too, we recommend early mobilisation and return to work.

Bed rest is also not necessary when back pain is caused by rigidity of the muscles. Resting would then only worsen the problem because the stiff muscles are no longer put to work.

If you must stay in bed, it is important not to get bored: radio, music, television, tablets, etc. can be of great help. Activities will be again possible as soon as you have sufficiently recovered to carry them out without pain. Even simple exercises can make a positive contribution to rehabilitation, for instance, making small circular movements with the foot, or moving the arms.

It is important to gradually reduce the period of bed rest. As soon as you can stand up comfortably for a few minutes, you should try to repeat that regularly. Gradually, you can then try to perform different positions and activities for a longer period of time. The idea is to let the back recover without any further injury taking place.

What position is the best?

If bed rest is prescribed for lower back pain, always discuss with your doctor or physical therapist what position is most comfortable, how you should move and how much activity is permitted. It is also advisable to thoroughly check your sleep system. This can be done by using the ten questions that you can find at the beginning of this book.

» Getting into and out of bed

Make sure you do not overload your back getting in and out of bed. Always avoid turning while in a bent position – a bent position followed by a twisting movement in your spinal column, increases the pressure on the inter-vertebral disc enormously.

If you lie on your back, the best way to get out of bed is as follows: pull up your knees and turn to the side. Then put your legs over the edge of the bed and push yourself up with your arms and elbows while using your legs as a lever (Figure 114).

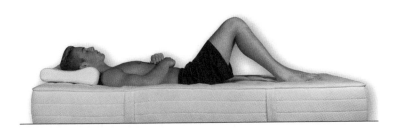

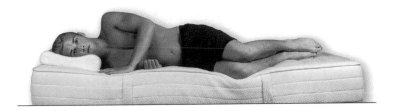

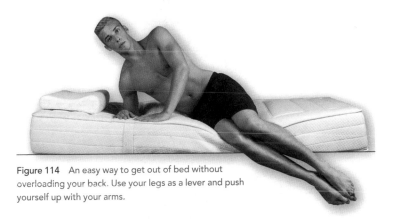

Figure 114 An easy way to get out of bed without overloading your back. Use your legs as a lever and push yourself up with your arms.

A safe way to get into bed without straining your back is: place your hands and one knee onto the bed, pull up the other knee to join it – a crawling motion – and then let your upper body sink by bending your arms (Figure 115). Pay attention to keeping your back straight the whole time and make sure it remains stable and doesn't twist.

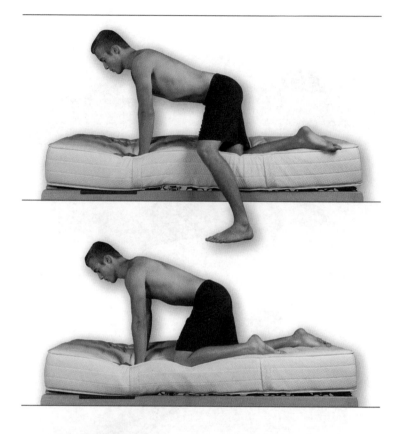

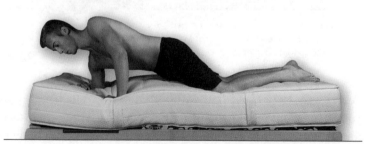

Figure 115 An easy way to get into bed. Above all, keep your back straight and bend your arms slowly.

» The astronauts' position

The resting position that physicians often recommend for patients with serious back symptoms is the so-called semi-Fowler's position: you lie on your back with hips and knees bent at a 45° angle, while the lower legs are supported (Figure 116). This position relaxes various muscles and promotes the return bloodflow to the heart. Because shoulders and hips are lying in the same horizontal plane, the spinal column is not being rotated.

It is noteworthy that the semi-Fowler's position pretty much coincides with the position that astronauts automatically assume when weightless. In zero gravity, all the joints go into a resting position.

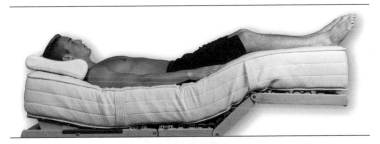

Figure 116   The astronauts' position or semi-Fowler's position.

People with an acute hernia are often advised to place the hips in a 90 degree angle when lying on the back. In this position, the iliopsoas muscle or internal hip flexor relaxes, the lower back curvature will flatten out and the inter-vertebral space increases. This increase of the inter-vertebral space causes a reduction in pressure in the inter-vertebral disc, and the nucleus will be sucked back into the inter-vertebral space. To what extent this mechanism effectively works is still unclear. This position does lead to slightly increased tension on the spinal cord and the posterior neural structures. The ligament that runs vertically along the rear of the vertebral body receives increased pressure and likewise exerts a force on the nucleus. The bulging connective tissue ring is thereby pulled tight, will bend away from the sciatic nerve and will exert less pressure on it (Figure 117).

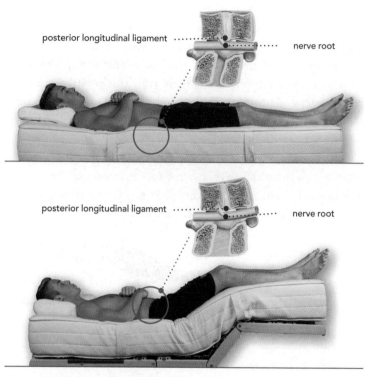

Figure 117 Thanks to the bent position, the rear side of the connective tissue ring is stretched, which can cause the bulging of the nerve root to subside. The effectiveness of this position is still being discussed.

TRYING OUT AND DELIBERATING

In summary: deciding which position is most favorable for you is something you can best discuss with your attending physician or physical therapist. Also try out which position is the least painful. This is often the right position for you.

Lying on your stomach is not advisable for the neck. The other sleep positions that we have described are suitable for back pain sufferers or for people who want to avoid back pain.

CHAPTER 10

Bed linen and hygiene

In this chapter we will talk about bed linen and what considerations you should bear in mind if you want to buy new sheets or a new duvet. We will also explain about house dust mites and reveal how these creatures can best be suppressed.

Bed linen is the last part of your sleep system, the part with which you have the closest contact. It protects your body and plays an important role in the regulation of moisture and heat in your bed.

By bed linen, we mean the mattress protector, the fitted sheet, the duvet, the duvet cover and possibly an upper flat sheet. With the exception of the duvet fillings, everything should preferably consist of 100 percent soft cotton.

THE DUVET

The duvet is the most important moisture buffer of your entire bed. It should maximally absorb and release the moisture that you evaporate during the night into the air. At the same time, it must store the heat, hence not to get too cold.

There is an enormous range of duvets on the market. We will provide a brief overview here.

The ticking of the duvet consists of 100 percent cotton or a blend of cotton and polyester, or microfibers and cotton. Preferably do not opt for polyester-cotton, because this combination scores least on moisture regulation.

The filling consists of either natural materials such as wool, cotton and down, or of solid or hollow synthetic fibers. Hollow synthetic fibers are more resilient and insulate better than solid fibers. Down can be used by itself, but is often mixed with feathers. The greater the percentage of down used, the lighter the duvet will be.

✗ Warmth classification or fill power

Every individual has a different need for warmth. This is why duvets are available in different warmth classes. This classification can give you something to go by if you are considering buying a new duvet. The following classification is often used in Western Europe:

- × Class 1: winter duvet; for cold rooms or if you opt for high heat insulation.
- × Class 2: average insulation; most commonly used.
- × Class 3: moderate insulation; for hot rooms or if you opt for low heat insulation.
- × Class 4: summer duvet; for hot nights.

A general used warmth classification in the UK is the Tog Rating.

A Tog is a unit of thermal resistance used to measure the power of insulation.

Duvets with a :

- × Tog rating 4–5   for summer use
- × Tog rating 6–10.5   for spring/autumn use
- × Tog rating 11–12   for those who prefer slightly more warmth
- × Tog rating above 12 for cold winter nights

We did not find a standardized US classification for the warmth nor for the weight of duvets.

The weight of a duvet is also a matter of personal preference. Some people really want to feel the weight of the duvet. For other people the duvet cannot be light enough. Duvets of a particular warmth class may vary considerably in weight because they are filled with a different material. For example wool is somewhat heavier than down. There are four weight classes in Western Europe. Because different types of filling materials have different insulation values, we can only compare the weights for each material with each other.

✖ How heavy?

Duvets are divided into four weight classes – the numbers below indicate how much a 55inch x 75inch duvet in those different classes weighs (best comparable to a full size duvet).
- × Super light: up to 1,200 grams/42 oz
- × Light: from 1,300 to 1,700 grams/46 to 60oz
- × Medium: from 1,800 to 2,400 grams/63 to 85 oz
- × Heavy: more than 2,500 grams/88 oz

Sometimes you can combine two duvets, so you get an extra thick one. For instance, super light combined with light yields the total comfort of heavy.

MAINTENANCE

Duvets require little maintenance. Just fluffing them up a bit every day and airing your room out keeps them in good condition. They can be washed at temperatures between 104 and 140°F. They can be aired outside. This is best done during warm dry weather, away from strong sunlight. The Deutsche Textilreinigungsverband (DTV) in Bonn recommends having duvets cleaned once a year by a specialized company.

DOWN OR SYNTHETIC?

There are so many differences between duvets with synthetic filling and duvets with down filling that we could write a whole book about that one subject alone. We do want to emphasize one important distinction here: there are fewer house dust mites in high-quality down duvets than in low-quality synthetic duvets. A low-quality synthetic duvet is generally produced in low-wage countries. It is filled with massive synthetic fibers, and has a cotton/polyester ticking that is not woven sufficiently dense.

A good down duvet has a very densely woven ticking of 100 percent cotton, a down percentage of 90 percent or more. Why the quality of a duvet is so important will be explained later in this chapter.

× Tip

Regardless of the type of duvet, it is important to air it out well in the morning and allow it to dry.

HOUSE DUST MITES AND ALLERGIES

More and more people suffer from allergies. Respiratory allergies (allergic rhinitis) have now become the most common form of allergy in the world and affect as many as 30 percent of adults and as many as 40 percent of children in the US; 5 to 12 percent of them suffer from allergic asthma. AR or allergic rhinitis, is estimated to affect nearly 1 in every 6 Americans. The US population is most commonly sensitized to grass pollen, dust mites and ragweed pollen. Almost 3% of all general practitioner consultations in the UK, for example, are about allergic rhinitis. This is partially due to our environment: scientists cite among other things air pollution, indoor smoking and an increased thermal insulation combined with inadequate ventilation. Research has been done for years on allergies arising from the sleeping environment and the sleep system. This has given rise to strategies to keep house mites and other micro-organisms in the bed under control.

Meet the enemy

House dust mites are tiny spiders. They have eight legs, and are less than 0.005 to 0.020 inches in size. They are found in large numbers in nearly all carpets, curtains, upholstered furniture, mattresses, pillows, duvets and the like.

Mites break down organic waste, especially flakes of human skin. We lose most of our dead skin flakes, about 0.8 inch a day, when we get dressed and undressed, and when we sleep. Older, moist skin flakes are often covered with molds. They break down the flakes into smaller pieces and thus making them more suitable as food and as a habitat for house dust mites. That explains why mold resistance is used as a strategy against the mites.

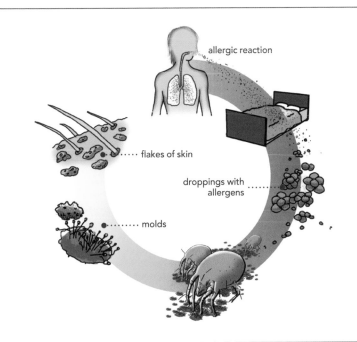

Figure 118   Molds enrich the flakes of skin as an optimal food source for the mites. The allergens that we inhale are being found on the droppings of the house dust mites.

The droppings of the mites are granules of fertilizer with a very small diameter, which, after drying out, easily disintegrate into even smaller particles. A protein in those droppings causes the well-known allergic reactions such as coughing, asthma, sneezing and watery eyes (Figure 118). This happens especially at night.

Allergic reactions occur only if there are many house dust mites who are getting enough food so that many droppings are released. The presence of a limited number of mites hardly constitutes a health risk.

Fighting the house dust mite

Completely eradicating house dust mites is virtually impossible, but fortunately it is not necessary. With the right interventions, we can already substantially limit exposure to the droppings and the associated allergic reactions. The most important measures you can take in the bedroom are: vacuuming, moisture control, use of adapted mattresses and bed linen, and finally optimising the relationship between heating and ventilation. Wash the bed linen preferably weekly at 140°F. Anyone who is allergic to house dust mites should preferably not make the bed themselves. It is also best not to get dressed and undressed in the bedroom, because in doing so you are spreading flakes of skin around the room.

The mite thrives at a temperature of 68 to 77°F and at a relative humidity of 70 to 75 percent. The best means of combating them is to keep the humidity in the bedroom under control. If the relative humidity is below 55 percent, the house dust mites get into trouble and below 45 percent they no longer occur. A combination of high temperatures – above 86°F – and low humidity is always fatal to a mite.

Mattresses and house dust mites

Mattresses are the favorite habitat of house dust mites. They find food here – through friction with the bedding, we lose our flakes of skin mainly in bed – and the accumulations of dust in which they love to live. Moreover, they are hard to chase away: you cannot easily just shove the whole mattress into the washing machine.

The creatures are found both inside the mattress and on the outside.

What can we do?

You can make life as unpleasant as possible for house dust mites by denying them moisture. It is therefore very important that you use good moisture-regulating bed linen. The higher the moisture buffering capacity of all the bed linen together, the lower the moisture load on the mattress, and the more difficult it gets for the house dust mite to survive. A good duvet is a must, because its ticking is so densely woven that mites cannot get through.

You would do best to opt for a mattress with a removable cover that is machine-washable at or above 140°F. The majority of such covers are filled with synthetic materials, because those you can wash at home. Covers filled with wool or other materials are best cleaned at a dry cleaner. After washing, most of the mites will be dead and the allergens will have been washed away. Finally, you can provide mattress cores, mattresses, pillows and even duvets with dust mite-resistant covers: they let air and moisture through, but block dust mites and their droppings.

Maintenance is easy. For maintenance follow the instructions on the label.

Mattresses that can be heated is also being addressed. A high longterm temperature is lethal to the mites. This is a promising idea, but the implementation is still in its infancy.

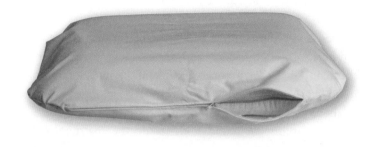

Figure 119   Pillows can also be provided with house dust mite-proof covers.

Bed linen and house dust mites

House dust mites can also be found in pillows and duvets. Pillows often contain the highest concentration because a lot of hair residue and flakes of skin can be found here.

Most people think that house dust mites flourish especially in bed linen with a natural filling such as down and feathers. A German study by Professor Hans W. Jürgens, however, shows that this is not entirely correct. The breeding grounds for the mite are flakes of human skin, not the cotton, wool, feathers, or down of the bedding.

It is also not true that down duvets are a breeding ground for mites. When you are lying under a duvet, it is too hot under the down for mites and when you are not lying under it, it gets too dry. Moreover, as mentioned, the 100 percent cotton covers of good down duvets are so densely woven that dust mites cannot get through. The advantages that down duvets offer a person – warming up quickly during sleep, rapid moisture removal during airing – are precisely those things that the house dust mite cannot stand.

It would be best to have down duvets dry-cleaned by a specialized down cleaning company. Cleaning these yourself or having them cleaned at the dry-cleaners is not recommended.

× Tips

Let's just view the practical tips at a glance:

- × Choose a duvet with a densely woven ticking that you can wash at a minimum of 140°F. Then dry thoroughly. Do this at least three times a year. Some models are protected against boiling temperatures and you can wash them at 194°F.
- × Wash pillowcases, mattress protectors, fitted sheets and duvet covers every week at 140°F.
- × If this is not enough, you can get bed linen fitted with allergen-proof barrier covers. It's best to replace mattresses older than five years and pillows older than three years. Also fit them immediately with allergen-proof barrier covers.
- × When buying a new mattress, opt for a mattress with a washable house dust mite-resistant outer cover.
- × Do not allow pets in the bedroom.
- × Vacuum all surfaces of upholstered furniture at least twice a week.
- × Reduce humidity by increasing ventilation. Use trickle vents in double glazing, or open windows. Use extract fans in bathrooms and kitchens.
- × Air the bed out well and make it just before you go to sleep.
- × Don't change clothes in the bedroom, and store clothes in closed closets.
- × Vacuum at least once a week. Use a HEPA filter: that stops nearly 100 percent of dust particles larger than 0.3 microns.

TEMPERATURE AND MOLD FORMATION

Molds are mostly found on walls, transitional areas between floors and walls, and transitional areas between ceilings and walls. They can mainly be seen in places where there is (excessive) moisture, combined with poor building construction such as inadequate ventilation facilities in bathrooms and kitchens.

Mold spores are very small and float around freely: so we breathe them in. They do not necessarily cause respiratory symptoms, but can make them worse. So moisture and mold do not belong in living areas. The main cause of problems with mold in **older** houses are poor building construction, uninsulated walls, leaky gutters and in particular the presence of thermal bridges.

The warmer the interior air, the more moisture it can absorb. If warm, moist air cools down rapidly, part of the moisture will condense or deposit, which can lead to mold formation. So make sure that the moist air can escape from the room. It is best to air out the room via an open window. This is best done in dry, cold or sunny weather. Be sure to prevent warm, moist air from flowing into your colder and drier bedroom because then the moisture in the air will partly condense there.

Above all, remember that in insufficiently heated bedrooms in **older homes,** the risk of moisture problems and mold formation increases. The minimum bedroom temperature should preferably be 59°F. If the temperature falls below this, the room needs to be ventilated more. Usually the opposite happens, with all consequences. Heat your house well, including the bedrooms, and don't let the bedroom cool off too much at night.

During sleep, the body produces heat that is partially transmitted and absorbed by the bed linen and the mattress. The mattress is warmer at the top than at the bottom. If, in the morning, you don't allow the bed to air out sufficiently, the warm air will only be able to move to the cooler bottom of the mattress, with a risk of condensation and mold formation. A mattress pad between the mattress and the bed base can reduce the risk of mold formation.

× Tips

- × In older houses, it is ideal to heat a bedroom at least once a week and afterwards let it ventilate. This will, of course, drive up the energy bill. This does not apply to newer homes.
- × Air the bedroom daily in dry weather, but preferably not in damp weather.
- × Limit the in-house production of moisture (showering, bathing, washing machines, airing cupboards, dryers...) and ensure proper discharge of the humid air. Check whether the ventilation facilities of the bathroom, kitchen and toilet are functioning properly and whether they are discharging enough air.

CHAPTER 11

The bedroom

Until now we have mainly discussed the influence of the sleep system on sleep quality. In this chapter we turn our attention to other factors that influence our night's sleep. There are many factors such as: temperature, ventilation, body movement, alcohol... But the biggest enemies of sleep are noise and light, so we'll start with those.

NOISE

We all know that we are woken by sudden, loud noises. This is a natural reflex of our body to verify that nothing is threatening our surroundings or that we have to run away or defend ourselves. Because we tend to be very alert during such an episode, it often takes a while before we can fall asleep again. A constantly high noise level – so, no peaks of noise – also has a negative impact on sleep quality. Studies in people living near a busy highway have proven that they move a lot more in their sleep and also wake up more often – women even more than men. Contrary to what we all think, we do not get used to that night-time noise: people who have been living next to a highway for years still suffer from a disturbed sleep pattern. The result is excessive daytime sleepiness and impaired mental and physical resistance.

LIGHT

The sleep-wake rhythm of our body follows a twenty-four hour pattern. A large number of body processes takes place according to that so-called circadian rhythm. Our body temperature, for instance, is the highest in the afternoon at around 4 p.m. and the lowest at night at around 4 a.m. The concentration of the growth hormone cortisol also follows such a diurnal rhythm: it plays a role in waking up, and reaches its highest concentration shortly after awakening. Cortisol is produced under the influence of light, so leaving a lamp on at night is actually not such a good idea. On the other hand, you should not darken your bedroom excessively. A moderate intensity of light in the early morning can increase the cortisol peak by 35 percent, with the result that your cardiovascular system and other organs are better prepared for a period of activity during the day.

TEMPERATURE

The regulation of our body temperature

Our body temperature is regulated by the hypothalamus, a part of the brain. Based on information that the hypothalamus receives from the central nervous system, the cardiovascular system and the skin, it will keep our temperature within safe limits, adapted to the circadian rhythm. This all acts as a negative feedback system: our body will cool off when the body temperature is increasing and warm up when the body temperature is decreasing. Every form of heat transfer happens in light of preserving our internal body temperature at around 98.6°F. Scientists call this homeothermy.

Body temperature and sleep

Temperature and sleep are tightly intertwined: they follow the same twenty-four hour rhythm and are synchronised with the alternation between day and night. Humans are diurnal animals: we sleep when it's dark and when our body temperature is low. We are awake when it's light and when our body temperature is high.

Figure 120 shows the connection between sleep-wake periods and temperature rhythms. We wake up because it gets light and because our body temperature rises. Conversely, we will become sleepy when it gets dark and our body temperature falls.

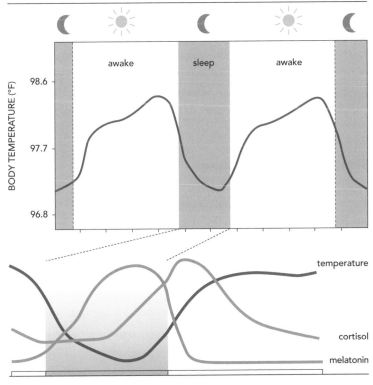

Figure 120   Schematic representation of three circadian rhythms. Melatonin values are very high during the night and very low at daytime. Cortisol values are the lowest at the beginning of the night and the highest after waking up. Our body temperature is the highest at the end of the day, decreases fast when falling asleep and reaches its lowest values about 3 hours before awakening.

That sleepy feeling is caused by the hormone melatonin. During the daytime melatonin breaks down under the influence of light, but when it gets dark, it slowly but surely increases.

Above we have already briefly discussed cortisol, another hormone that plays an important role in our sleep-wake system. The lowest concentration of cortisol shows when falling asleep and during the first five hours of sleep. Then the concentration gradually builds up again – also under the influence of light – until we wake up. It is therefore sometimes referred to as the *wake-up hormone*. As soon as we are awake, the cortisol level begins to drop gently, and the cycle starts all over again.

We mostly fall asleep while our body temperature is decreasing – the shortest time it takes to fall asleep coincides with the lowest body temperature. Conversely, we almost never fall asleep when our body temperature is rising. The underlying mechanism that controls the core body temperature is dependent on the skin temperature.

Skin and bed temperature

For a large part of the day, the exterior of our body – our skin – is colder than the inside: usually at around 82.4°F. Towards the evening, however, the body begins to move heat from the inside to the outside. The skin temperature increases, and the distinction between core body temperature and skin temperature blurs.

When we lie down in bed, the skin temperature rises even further, due to, among other things, the thermal insulation capacity of our sleep system. At this point, the bed temperature – the overall temperature under the sheets – starts to play an important role. If it remains between 80.6 and 84.2°F, the skin temperature will not go higher or lower – it will remain at a constant 95°F, which is perfect.

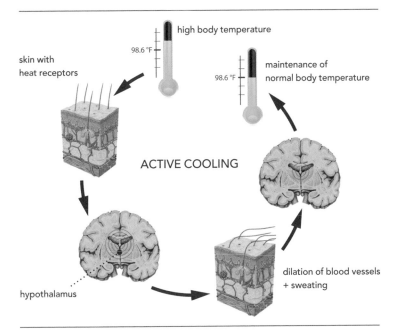

skin with
heat receptors

high body temperature

98.6 °F

98.6 °F

maintenance of
normal body temperature

ACTIVE COOLING

hypothalamus

dilation of blood vessels
+ sweating

Figure 121   Simplified representation of the role of the hypothalamus as 'control center' of the body temperature. When body and/or skin temperature rise sharply, heat-sensitive neurons in the hypothalamus activate the dilation of the blood vessels and sweat secretion. Thanks to this heat loss, the body temperature decreases, and the activity of the hypothalamus decreases.

But usually, the bed temperature will begin to rise somewhat. The **heat receptors** in our skin will send information to the heat sensitive neurons in the hypothalamus about this, allowing them to 'regulate' the situation. Our body begins to cool off by dilating blood vessels and sweating, and this way the skin temperature is kept at 95°F. Scientists speak of the negative feedback system. We call this 'active cooling'.

The feedback system works perfectly – until the bed temperature reaches 93.2°F. At that moment, it will become very uncomfortable. Our skin temperature will rise above 96.8°F, and we will begin to toss and turn. The proportion of deep sleep will decrease, with the result that we will not feel well the following day.

In a typical bedroom in Western Europe and the US, we will not often see a bed temperature below 80.6°F. This is fortunate, because if it does happen, our body will again take measures to maintain our temperature. This time, it is the **cold receptors** in the skin that inform the **cold-sensitive neurons** in the hypothalamus about the situation. The blood vessels constrict, we begin to shiver, we move more often, our metabolic activity increases... We call this negative feedback system 'active heating'. In extreme situations, these are all things that are not conducive to a good night's sleep – anyone who, while camping, has experienced a cold night in a sleeping bag that is too thin, will know what we are talking about.

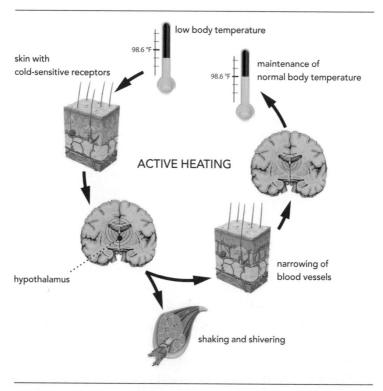

Figure 122 When body and/or skin temperature drops sharply, cold-sensitive neurons in the hypothalamus activate narrowing of the blood vessels (heat retention) and activate the muscles to produce heat. This results in an increase in body temperature and this will suppress the neurons in the hypothalamus.

There is a clear relationship between skin temperature and being asleep or being awake. A warm skin – up to 95°F – seems to promote sleep, and to decrease alertness. A cold skin seems to counteract sleep and to promote alertness. We suspect that the increasing skin temperature in the evening increases the activity of the warm-sensitive neurons in the hypothalamus, and it is these signals from the warm-sensitive neurons that promote sleep.

The hypothalamus is not only involved in the timing of the sleep-wake rhythm, but also seems to be the main neural network for the regulation of body temperature.

In order to be able to fall asleep quickly and to attain a good sleep quality, it is also important that our 'extremities' are not too cold in during wintertime (especially our feet) and are not too hot during summertime (especially our head).

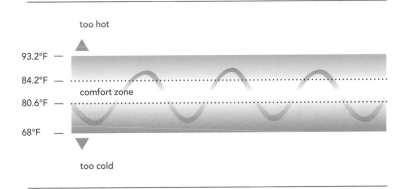

Figure 123   Within the comfort or thermo-neutral zone, the skin temperature remains fairly constant at around 95°F. Our body thus hardly has to actively cool down or heat up.

Maintening an optimal bed temperature depends strongly on bed linen, pyjamas and sleep system. Even our bed partner has some influence. He or she also radiates heat, and his/her movements may possibly disturb the temperature equilibrium. On average, women appear to prefer warmer temperature, men prefer cooler temperature. There might also be preferential differences between Northern and Southern Europeans.

The temperature of the bedroom

It is often said that the ideal bedroom temperature is between 60.8 to 64.4°F, but this is not always true. Factors such as age, gender, sleep habits and bed linen play a big role. The optimal bedroom temperature for a young man lying under a thick down duvet, could be 50°F; for an older woman under a thin sheet, would this bedroom temperature perhaps more likely be 75.2°F. In addition, our temperature regulation system functions differently during the winter than during the summer.

But very generally, we can say: if the ambient temperature in the winter drops below 53.6°F, either our body will cool off too much or we will have to cover up so thickly that we will experience the extra bed linen as unpleasant. The phases of deep sleep and REM sleep will reduce. The total sleeping time may also be shortened, and insomnia may increase.

✗ Tip

Make sure that, during wintertime, the bedroom temperature does not drop below 60.8°F.

On the other hand, an excessively high ambient temperature during summer – above 75.2°F – can cause the bed temperature to increase. The body heat is dissipated more slowly, and the skin and body temperature will increase too much. The reduction in body temperature which is so essential for sleep, is compromised. In addition, the humidity of the sleep system will go up, resulting in damp skin, which feels very uncomfortable.

✗ Tip

Make sure that, during summertime, the bedroom temperature preferably does not exceed 76.8°F.

Room temperatures around 53.6 to 62.6°F can generally be well tolerated if we have a good sleep system with adapted bed linen.

In bed, we cool off mostly through our head, and also a little through our hands and feet. Lower bedroom temperatures – but not lower than 53.6°F – will accelerate the cooling of the head, which promotes falling asleep and has a positive effect on deep sleep. Hands and feet need to be warm just before going to bed, because then the blood vessels dilate and the body heat can be removed more easily. That also makes it easier to fall asleep.

Temperature and REM sleep

Research has shown that there is a connection between ambient temperature, bed temperature, REM cycle duration and REM sleep.

During REM sleep the thermal regulation of our body discontinues. The thermostat no longer works. Researchers describe this phenomenon as a decoupling of our central control system in the hypothalamus from both the spinal cord and our brainstem.

We can no longer control our temperature by shivering or sweating, and therefore, the skin and body temperatures begins to vary along with the ambient temperature.

In an extremely hot or cold environment, our body cools off or heats up too much, which according to some researchers should provoke a wake-up stimulus. Because the periods of REM sleep in the first part of the night are of relatively short duration – from 10 to 15 minutes – we used to think that the effect on body and skin temperatures would be small. Recent research shows however that even small changes in skin temperature can have a relatively large impact on sleep structure. During the second part of the night, when we have more REM sleep, the sleeper will experience even more discomfort as a result of it.

The temperature regulation is disturbed, but not completely switched off! A study by Alain Muzet has revealed that at bedroom temperatures above 77°F, the REM cycle time was about 24 minutes shorter. The REM cycle is the period between the end of one and the beginning of the following stage of REM. A shorter REM cycle therefore means that the proportion of deep sleep diminishes. This is not so good: we will feel less well rested the next day (Figure 124).

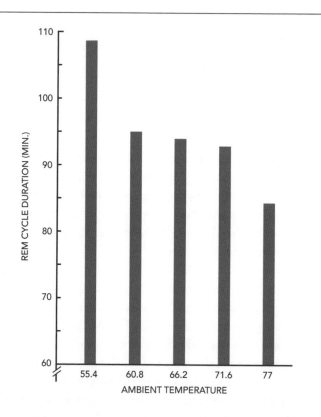

Figure 124 Influence of ambient temperature (°F) on the REM cycle duration (in minutes).

At a high temperature, we start tossing and sweating, as we have seen above, and our metabolic activity increases. When the temperature drops, our metabolism slows down and our REM cycle duration increases. This could indicate that it is better to sleep in a cool room than in a warm room.

The effect of heat on sleep

A warm and humid environment reduces the proportion of deep sleep and REM sleep, as we have seen above, and increases and extends the number of awake periods. The negative effect of humid heat is bigger at the beginning of sleep.

However, recent studies in elderly people show that a slight increase in temperature of the skin – within the limits of the level of comfort – increases the proportion of deep sleep and increases the total sleep duration. Even healthy people without sleep problems fall asleep faster if the skin temperature rises slightly in advance. A warm bath, fifteen minutes in the sauna or a hot-water bottle will therefore certainly help you to fall asleep.

Not every method is equally successful. An electric blanket appears to disturb sleep. The most likely explanation is that it emits heat for too long and as a result, also forces the core body temperature to rise. As we have seen above, it is very difficult to fall asleep when the body temperature is rising.

The trick is to ensure that the skin temperature raises slightly, but certainly not the body temperature. In other words, we seek a balance and we all know that balances don't last forever. These methods will therefore primarily promote falling asleep and will improve sleep during the first part of the night.

The effect of cold on sleep

So, in wintertime, heat – within the limits of the comfort zone – will primarily have a positive effect during the first part of the night. Cold will mainly influence the second part of the night, when REM sleep is dominant. With colder bed temperature we see that people wake up more often and exhibit less REM sleep.

If you have a good heat insulating mattress and use heat insulating bed linen, low bedroom temperatures will scarcely have any impact on the bed temperature and therefore on sleep.

During summer, when the bedroom temperature often exceeds 68°F, retaining the temperature within the limits of the comfort zone is not so simple. People living in a hot climate will probably have already experienced the advantage of air-conditioning.

We do it ourselves

We do have to ask ourselves an important question: is it necessary to influence the skin temperature in order to promote sleep? Based on video analyses we can say that during short waking moments, people do all kinds of temperature-regulating things, for instance, they remove the duvet to expose the legs to a cooler environment, or cover themselves up better to get warmer. This all can happen consciously or unconsciously.

Unconsciously, we take other heat-regulating actions. For instance, with higher bed temperatures, the ratio of lying on one's side to lying on one's back increases, probably because this way, the contact surface between the body and the (warm) mattress is smaller. We must again conclude that sleep is something active, and that the bed linen and the mattress certainly affect our sleeping positions.

HUMIDITY IN THE BEDROOM

The degree of humidity in a bedroom is very variable and can reach percentages above 70 percent. **Too much humidity** around your sleep system will shorten the life of the mattress and increase the survival of dust mites, as we saw in Chapter 10. If the humidity gets too high the body will also feel damp and warm, which undermines the quality of sleep.

But we should also try to avoid **too little humidity**. When the weather is conducive to open the bedroom windows, the indoor humidity is approximately equal to the outdoor humidity. When we are not able to ventilate the room enough, the water vapor that we evaporate during sleep generally increases the indoor humidity. For that reason, try to keep the moisture balance under control by airing regularly. Ideally, the degree of relative humidity in the bedroom should remain below 70 percent.

× Tips

We conclude this book with a few tips for a good night's sleep, based on common sense, scientific research and our own personal experience.

- × Regularity is the golden rule. Go to bed at a fixed time; get up at a fixed time. A fixed sleep-wake rhythm boosts sleep quality.
- × Sleep long enough. For an adult human being, that is seven to eight hours. Above the age of fifty, the average sleep time may drop to fewer than six hours, but short daytime naps usually ensure that the total amount of sleep is sufficient and the proportion of deep sleep remains the same. Sleep deprivation leads to physical symptoms such as high blood pressure, obesity and so on.
- × Illuminate the room in the morning when getting up: sufficient light helps our biological clock.

- × Conversely, arrange for subdued lighting at night before bedtime and don't leave a light on in the bedroom at night. Naturally, that also means that you do not leave the TV on if you have one in your bedroom. If you cannot darken the bedroom enough, it might be necessary to use an eye shade.
- × Staying in bed too long – which for most people is longer than eight hours – can worsen problems with falling asleep and staying asleep through the night.
- × Ensure comfortable sleep accommodation with good light exclusion, good sound insulation, and the right temperature.
- × Go to bed with the intention to sleep – with a relaxed body and mind. During the hour before bedtime you should avoid doing things that put your brain to work (intellectual work, financial matters...) or increase your adrenaline level (games, exciting films or TV episodes...). Also, try not to brood about problems at work or in your family. Make the hour before you go to bed a relaxation period, with activities such as reading a book, listening to relaxing music, taking a hot bath.
- × Do not panic if you can't fall asleep immediately. It may help if you get up after twenty minutes and do some relaxation exercises: consciously regulating your breathing also has a calming effect. Feeling relaxed results in slower and more regular breathing which can help you fall asleep. Continuing to breath like that can help you fall asleep.
- × If you suffer from a sleep disorder, avoid turning your bedroom into a work- or dining room or a TV corner.
- × Avoid stimulating or irritating foods and/or stimulants. No coffee, tea, coke or strong alcoholic beverages just before bedtime. Alcohol makes you fall asleep faster, but it also ensures that you sleep less deeply and wake up sooner.
- × Good things to consume before bedtime are one glass of wine, dairy products, chicken, nuts, malt products and vitamin B.

- × Keep at least a period of three hours between dinner and bedtime, otherwise your body will need to invest too much energy in digestion and your sleep will be disturbed.
- × Have a light meal in the evening and avoid spicy foods. Chocolate is not recommended either.
- × So don't overeat, but don't go to bed feeling hungry either. If you're still feeling hungry, you could have a light snack that is high in carbohydrates such as a cookie, cereal with milk, or a slice of wholeweat bread.
- × Make sure you regularly engage in physical exercise, ideally every day, before dinner, and at the latest two hours before bedtime.
- × Make sure you have a good bed. It should be one of your most precious possessions, because it plays a key role in your well-being and your physical health.

Hopefully you now have a good understanding of the conditions a bed should meet, and a clearer picture of the sleep system that suits you best.

Best of luck!

The bed of the future

In the previous chapters, you discovered how your body and your bed have an influence on each other and how important it is to choose the right bed system. Throughout the years (and centuries) our beds have undergone a huge evolution. This development is still an ongoing process. Custom8, a spin-off of the Catholic University of Leuven (KUL), is researching how our bed can even be improved in the future. We will provide an overview of the state of affairs here.

A BIOMECHATRONIC SLEEPING DEVICE

Whenever greater optimisations are needed than the classical sciences are able to accomplish, new sciences are arising. For example, thermodynamics, which arose during the industrial revolution out of the need to make steam engines more efficient, and mechatronics, which, as an engineering science, burgeoned from the need to describe mechanical systems that were driven by computer-controlled electronics. So too, is biomechanics reaching its limits to design passive sleep systems to keep up with the growing demands of the ever more aware human being. The same way as cars have evolved from a classic piece of mechanics into efficient computer-controlled machines, so too are classic beds going to give way to sleeping devices that adapt to the physical desires and needs of the user. A bed is thus gradually evolving into a biomechatronic sleep device.

WHICH SLEEP FACTORS SHOULD BE IMPROVED?

In order to develop a sleep system that can offer more than a classic passive bed, it is important to identify the factors that may or may not positively affect the quality of sleep. These factors may be of an environmental (such as light interference or excess noise), a biomechanical (lying position, sensation of comfort, pressure distribution), a psychological (e.g. stress) or a medical (snoring, apnoea) nature. The lying position, for instance, is one factor that determines the quality of sleep, but which, due to the very different compression profiles in lateral and supine positions may only be capable of restricted optimisation by a passive sleep system and as a result is perfectly eligible to be actively corrected during sleep.

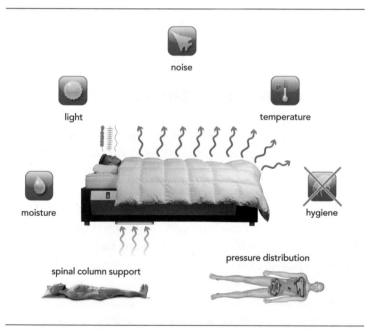

Figure 125 The bed of the future is a biomechatronic sleep device that adjusts itself to environmental factors (light, noise) and the microclimate close to the skin and that makes use of cutting-edge technology in order to measure and adjust parameters and physiological sleep processes that are unique to the body.

HOW SHOULD ONE MEASURE?

To actively optimize sleep quality, it is necessary to monitor one or more sleep factors during sleep at regular intervals. An active sleep system always contains a measuring system that measures the desired factors during sleep. Sometimes sleep factors can be measured directly (e.g. temperature, light, sound), but usually the measurement must be done in a roundabout way (according to the lying position, heart rate or breathing) and a biomechanical, mathematical or statistical model forms the basis of the measurement.

Therefore the lying position can only be accurately determined based on a measurement of the deformation of the mattress surface on one hand, and on the other hand by a biomechanical model of the human being with the body parameters of the sleeper.

It is thus not only essential to perform an accurate measurement, but there must also be sufficient additional information in order to arrive at the desired factor through calculations. An insufficiently accurate measurement combined with a lack of essential additional model information is very often the source of erroneous interpretations of the events during sleep.

An example of this is the pressure measurement. Whereas an accurate pressure measurement is effective for mapping the distribution of pressure over the mattress surface, it is totally inadequate for calculating the spinal support. Moreover, a perfect mathematical description of the physical properties of the bed materials is unattainable in any case.

HOW CAN SLEEP QUALITY BE ACTIVELY IMPROVED?

To be of value in an active sleep system, the measurement that brings one or more aspects of sleep quality into the picture must be evaluated on the basis of scientific criteria. This evaluation is important in order to estimate what adjustments the sleep system must make for the sleeper in the measured situation to sleep better. In the case of a lying position, there will be an evaluation of the extent to which the measured position deviates from the optimal lying position. Then the corrections that the sleep system should perform to achieve this correct sleeping position are calculated. The active sleep system will be equipped in this case with zones, the firmness of which can be soundlessly adjusted during sleep. By adjusting the firmness in different zones, corrections to positions may be carried out, such as the position of the shoulders when lying on one's side, supporting the waist, correcting the pelvic tilt and so on.

EXAMPLES OF ACTIVE CONTROL

Other examples of active control revolve around climate control in the sleep system to increase the sleeping comfort throughout the seasons. Both the temperature and the humidity in the sleep system must be actively controlled to avoid mold and dust mites. By controlling the temperature near the skin, the behavior conducive to falling asleep could be increased. Based on measured skin temperatures during sleep, an automatic heating or cooling system might also be useful and perhaps in the future the flow of fresh air in our bedroom will occur through the bed system.

Another promising example is the complete or partial elimination of obstructive sleep apnoea by targeted stiffening of the zone of kyphosis (the convex curvature at the level of the thoracic vertebrae) in the supine position.

Still other applications include detecting sleep phases using statistical calculations based on the extent of movement, breathing and changes of body position. Active control of the illumination of the room can then ensure that the sleeper is awakened slowly and in the right stage of sleep.

Acknowledgments

A big thank you to everyone who made this book possible, in particular:

× Editor **Wim Heyvaert**, for the permanent quest for the right words in 'plain language'.
× Graphics experts **Marc Jacops** and **Frank Geisler** for their ability to make the exciting world of human anatomy, and in particular the structure of the spinal column, clearer for the reader.
× **Jens Trappeniers** as a model for the beautiful photos.
× **Chris Raets and Martine Derveaux** for the work behind the scenes.
× Last but not least: **my family** for their support and patience.

Also, my sincere thanks to the team of professors and experts for the useful tips, comments and support from the academic world in reading the book. In particular:

× Prof. Dr. **Gaëtane Stassijns**, attached to the Faculty of Medicine and Health Sciences and a physician in the Department of Physical Medicine and Rehabilitation at the University Hospitals of Antwerp (www.uza.be).
× **Hilde Verbiest**, occupational therapist attached to the Department of Physical Medicine and Rehabilitation at the University Hospitals of Antwerp (www.uza.be).
× Prof. Dr. **Simon Brumagne**, attached to the Department of Rehabilitation Sciences of the Faculty of Kinesiology and Rehabilitation Sciences of the Catholic University of Leuven, Belgium and physiotherapist in the Department of Physical Medicine and Rehabilitation - CERM University Hospitals Leuven Gasthuisberg Campus (www.uzleuven.be).

× Prof. Dr. **Ton Coenen**, Emeritus Professor of Sleep Studies at Radboud University Nijmegen (www.ru.nl).
× Prof. Ir. **Bart Haex**, attached to the Biomechanics Department of the Faculty of Engineering Sciences of the Catholic University of Leuven (KUL) (www. mech.kuleuven.be).
× The engineers of **Custom8**, spin-off of the Catholic University of Leuven (KUL) specialising in biomedical and technological innovations (www.cus-tom8.be).
× Ir. **Atze Boerstra,** engineer and expert in the field of indoor climate and air quality associated with BBA Indoor Environment BV The Hague (www.binnenmilieu.nl).

May this book be a source of inspiration for the many scientists of any discipline whatsoever, who are involved in sleep research and research into the pathogenesis and treatment of back and neck problems. The multidisciplinary approach of these health problems and the cooperation with product developers and engineers should enable us to develop better sleep systems for the human beings on this planet.

Explanatory glossary

Allergens
Substances foreign to the body which cause allergic symptoms in individuals susceptible to them.

Annulus fibrosus
The outer part of the inter-vertebral disc, consisting of several layers of fibrocartilage collagen, which connects two vertebrae with each other.

Arterioles
Small arteries.

Arthrosis
Arthrosis is a collective term for a wide variety of diseases of the joints, all with the same result which is an often painful degeneration of the joints. It is an abnormal condition of the joints whereby loss of cartilage, hardening of the bone underneath the cartilage, and a varying degree of inflammation in the joint capsule are found. Small bone spurs can also emerge at the edge of the joint.

Atrophy
Deterioration of the nutritional status of organs, making them shrink or shrivel.

Bedridden
Restrained to bed.

Biological clock
Innate mechanism whereby all kinds of bodily functions take place with a certain periodicity, such as the sleep-wake rhythm.

Body Mass Index (BMI)
Index which represents a certain relationship between height and weight in a person, and which is an indicator for over- or under-weight. The value of the index is equal to the weight of the body (in kilograms) divided by the square of the height (in metres).

Brainstem
Lower part of the brain that is connected to the spinal cord.

Bronchitis
Inflammation of the bronchi in the lungs, called bronchial tubes, at the level of the branchings of the trachea and alveoli.

Bronchus
Airway in the respiratory track that conducts air to the lungs.

Canalis vertebralis
Spinal canal or central canal of the spinal cord (canalis centralis).

Capillaries
The finest branches of blood vessels.

Capsule
(Joint) capsule.

Cardiovascular
Relating to the heart and blood vessels.

Cartilage
Elastic structures that cover articular processes.

Cauda equina
Name for the spinal roots which are suspended like a tail (horse's tail) from the lower portion of the spinal cord, and emerge two-by-two from the spinal column.

Central nervous system
Part of the nervous system consisting of the brain and the spinal cord, from where – as from a centre – the nerves emerge.

Cerebellum
Part of the brain situated behind and below the cerebrum.

Cerebrospinal fluid (CSF)
Brain and spinal fluid, the liquid which is situated between the soft membrane and the arachnoid membrane of the brain and spinal cord and which also fills the brain cavities.

Cerebrum
Largest part of the brain with convolutions and grooves on its surface.

Cervical
In orthopaedics, relating to the cervical spine.

Circadian Rhythm
Biological rhythm in which the cycle lasts approximately one day. It is also referred to as a 24-hour rhythm or sleep-wake rhythm or cycle. The rhythm is controlled by the biological clock.

Collagen
Protein component of connective tissue fibers, cartilage and bone.

Connective tissue
Biological tissue that supports, connects, or separates different types of tissues and organs in the body.

Cortisol
Hormone produced in the adrenal cortex according to a circadian rhythm. When waking up, more cortisol is released.

Creep
Process in which elongation of connective tissue occurs.

Deformation
Distortion.

Degeneration
Morbid changes in the cells or the tissue, causing their quality to deteriorate; wear and tear (often under the influence of age).

Dehydration
Withdrawal or loss of moisture from the tissues.

Density
Density or more precisely, the volumetric mass density, of a substance is its mass per unit volume. Mathematically = ounces/cubic inch.

Dermatophagoides
House dust mite, a pteronyssinus mite common in house dust which secretes an allergen that causes allergic reactions such as wheezing.

Diffusion
Mixture of solutes with solvents or liquids with other liquids, when they come into contact with each other.

Discosis (degenerative disc disease or chondrosis inter-vertebralis)
Degeneration of the inter-vertebral disc.

Discus inter-vertebralis

Inter-vertebral disc, a deformable disc located between two vertebrae. It consists of a layer of connective tissue fibers (annulus fibrosus), around a gelatinous core (nucleus pulposus).

Dural

Relating to the hard brain membrane called the dura mater. *See:* dura mater.

Dura mater

The outer of the three meninges, the hard membrane covering the brain and the spinal cord. The brain as well as the spinal cord is surrounded by three membranes, namely, the inner or soft membrane (pia mater), the middle or arachnoid membrane (arachnoidea) and the outer or hard membrane (dura mater), which encloses the spinal cord and the brain.

Electroencephalogram (EEG)

A measurement of the electrical activity associated with brain activity.

Electromyogram (EMG)

A measurement of the electrical activity associated with muscle movement.

Electroculogram (EOG)

A measurement of the electric activity associated with eye movements.

Epidemiology

The science relating to frequency and spreading of diseases in association with their underlying causes and origins.

Extension

Bending backwards.

Extension load
Putting strain on spinal column structures when bending backwards or stretching.

Facet joints
The most posterior joints by which the vertebrae are interconnected.

Facet pain
Joint capsule pain.

Fibrosis
Increase of connective tissue in an organ.

Flattening
Reduction of the lordosis. *See:* lordosis.

Flexion
Bending forward.

Flexion strain
Putting strain on spinal column structures when bending forward.

Inter-vertebral foramen
Inter-vertebral opening, cavity between two vertebrae along which the spinal cord nerves leave the spinal column.

Joint protrusion (articular process)
Bony protrusion on the vertebra with which the connection is made with the adjacent vertebrae. Each vertebra has four joint projections, left and right, as well as above and below. Two by two, these projections form a small joint with the protrusions of the adjacent vertebrae, so that the vertebrae can move relative to each other. These small joints are called facet joints.

Functional unit
See: spinal column segment.

Ganglion spinale
(dorsal root ganglion or spinal cord ganglion)
Thickening in the course of a nerve with accumulation of neuronal cell bodies.

Growth hormone
Hormone that stimulates cell metabolism of all tissues and stimulates body growth by activating cell division and cell growth.

Headboard
An uprigh unit of wood, metal, plastic or upholstered material, to be attached at the head of a bed, usually with the bed frame.

HEPA filter
HEPA is the abbreviation for High Efficiency Particulate Air and is applicable to a specific type of air filter which keeps back 99.99 percent of all dust particles larger than 0.3 microns.

Hernia (hernia nuclei pulposi)
Bulging of the soft core of the inter-vertebral disc (nucleus pulposus) by the outermost torn connective tissue rings (annulus fibrosus), whereby pressure may develop on the roots of the spinal nerves.

High resilience
Highly flexible, an indication of a type of soft polyurethane foam.

Homeostasis
The being in balance of all the functions in the body.

Hormone
Substance formed by a gland and transported via the blood to organs or target cells upon which it has a specific effect.

Hyperextension
Overstretching a joint.

Hyperlordosis
An excessive lumbar curvature, which may give rise to chronic back pain.

Hypertrophy
Strong development of tissues or organs.

Hypnogram
Sleep curve that records the depth of sleep.

Hypothalamus
Part of the intermediate brain that affects the secretion of hormones and contains the thirst, hunger and temperature centres area.

Iliopsoas muscle
Internal hip flexor.

Inhibition
Restraint, obstruction; suppression of an impulse.

Innervation
Nerve function, the influence of the nerves on the operations of the organs, for instance on the muscle activity.

Insomnia
Sleeplessness; insomnia refers to persistent sleep problems such as disturbance falling asleep and sleeping through the night, associated with difficulties during the day.

Intradiscal pressure (IDP)
The pressure in the inter-vertebral disc.

Ischaemia
Decreased blood flow through obstruction of the blood supply.

Kyphosis
Backward (physiological) curvature of the spinal column (convex back); normally occurring in the thoracic section of the spinal column.

Latency (sleep onset latency)
Period of time between waking and sleeping.

Lesion
Harm, injury, damage.

Ligaments
The bands of connective tissue that tie the vertebral joints together. Short bands (ligamentum flavum, ligamentum supraspinale, ligamentum interspinale) run from one vertebra to the other. Long bands run along the entire spinal column, at the front (ligamentum longitudinale anterius or anterior longitudinal ligament) and at the back (ligamentum longitudinale posterius or posterior longitudinal ligament). The main function of the ligaments is to hold the vertebrae together.

Liquor (cerebrospinalis)
Liquid found within the dura mater, around the brain and spinal cord.

Lordosis
Forward (physiological) curvature of the spinal column (concave back), occurring normally in the cervical and lumbar sections of the spinal column.

Lower back pain
See: lumbago.

Lumbago
Medical term for (mostly) acute lower back pain which usually tends to manifest on one side of the lumbar area.

Lumbar
Relating to the lumbar spine, the lower back.

Lumbar spine
The part of the spinal column located at the lower back.

Lymphedema
Lymphedema is a condition of localized fluid retention and tissue swelling caused by a compromised lymphatic system, which normally returns interstitial fluid to the thoracic duct, then the bloodstream.

Mattress protector
A mattress protector, common on the Continent, made of a twill fabric called molton.

Medulla spinalis
Spinal cord.

Melatonin
Hormone produced by the pineal gland, the production of which is directly linked to exposure to light. In the presence of bluish (day) light, the production is inhibited. If the exposure to light decreases, the natural production starts up again. For the body, this is the signal to reduce the day's activities and to prepare for the night.

Metabolism
The collective chemical changes that take place in the organism in order to build it up and maintain it and also the conversion (decomposition) of living matter to simple substances to be excreted.

Metabolic substances
Substances that play an indispensable role in the metabolic process.

Motion segment
The smallest physiological motion unit of the spine exhibit bio-mechanical characteristics similar to those of the entire spine, also called functional spinal unit. It consists of two adjacent vertebrae, the inter-vertebral disc and all adjoining ligaments between them and excludes other connecting tissues such as muscles.

Negative feedback
System in which the increase of certain substances will inhibit the production of its own, and wherein the decrease of those substances will stimulate its production.

Nerves
Collection of nerve bundles consisting of nerve fibers, and surrounded by a connective tissue sheath.

Nerve root
Branch of the spinal nerve that begins at the level of the spinal cord.

Nervus ischiadicus
Sciatic nerve: the term 'sciatica' is derived from this.

Neural
Belonging to the nerve tissue; related to a nerve.

Neurology
The knowledge of the somatic diseases of the nervous system and their treatment.

Nociception
The detection of harmful external influences, usually through pain sensation.

Nucleus pulposus
The jelly-like core of the inter-vertebral disc.

Oedema
Accumulation of fluid in tissues, leading to a swelling.

Osteophyte
Exostosis. A bony growth, usually pointed, that forms by prolonged irritation of periosteum (vascular connective tissue around bones) or ligament.

Peripheral nervous system
The nervous system outside the central nervous system, network of nerves that connects the brain and spinal cord to the rest of the body; includes cranial and spinal nerves and two peripheral cords.

Physiological lordosis
Natural (normal) lordosis.

Plexus
Literally, braid; network or web of nerves or blood vessels.

Plexus brachialis
Brachial plexus; nerve plexus of branches of the lower cervical and upper thoracic nerves.

Polyether
A synthetic foam, which may or may not be CFC-free, foamed with a specific cell structure.

Polyurethane (PU)
PU is the collective name for various kinds of soft synthetic foams which are made from petroleum.

Prolapse

The first stage of a hernia whereby the fibers of the connective tissue rings are stretched, with the result that the material from the core can bulge out.

Proprioception

The deep muscle feeling that is triggered by receptors in muscles and joints.

Protrusion

Bulging; the second stage of a herniated disc, in which fibers of the connective tissue ring tear, allowing the material from the core to protrude further. As a result, pressure on pain-sensitive structures can arise. Only the outermost fibers of the connective tissue ring prevent the material from the core from making its way to the outside.

Psoas position

Lying position used for acute back symptoms; in supine position with the legs bent at an angle of approximately 45° at the pelvis and at the knee, so that the lower legs are supported. This will relax the iliopsoas muscle (internal hip flexor) and reduce the pressure on the intervertebral discs. Also known as semi-Fowler's position.

Radiation pain

Pain that travels the length of a nerve – for instance, down an entire arm or leg, for instance, from a nerve to the nerve branches, down an entire arm or leg.

Radicular

Related to the spinal root (radix).

Radicular pain

Pain radiating along the path of the nerve roots from the neck region to the elbows and even into the hands, or from the lumbar region to the legs and feet.

Receptor
Specialised cell that can register a specific stimulus and convert this stimulus to an impulse.

Reflex
Involuntary response to certain stimuli.

Rehydration
Re-uptake of moisture or elimination of dehydration through moisture supply.

Relative humidity (RH)
RH indicates as a percentage how much water vapor the air contains relative to the maximum amount of water vapor. Indoors, the RH is usually 40 to 60 percent.

Relaxation
Release of stress. Relaxation exercises are a type of physical exercise intended to help the muscles and the mind relax. They make use of deep breathing techniques as well as stretching and releasing specific muscle groups.

REM
Rapid Eye Movement, the phase of sleep characterised by rapid movements of the eyes.

REM cycle duration
Duration measured from the beginning of a REM phase until the beginning of the next REM phase.

REM sleep
Phase of sleep characterised by rapid eye movements (REM) and dreams.

Sacrum

The lowest part of the spinal column which consists of five vertebrae fused together to which then ultimately the coccyx (tailbone) is secured. By means of two joints, the sacrum is very firmly attached to the pelvis. These are the so-called sacroiliac joints.

Segment

See: spinal column segment.

Sensors

Collective name for various specialized cells and nerve endings located in or just under the skin, which send signals to the brain about the sensation that they are observing.

Sciatica

Sciatica is the pain caused by irritation of the sciatic nerve. This is a very thick nerve which originates at the level of the last vertebra and which runs along the buttock to the leg. Pain may radiate from the back into a leg when a herniated inter-vertebral disc compresses one of the branches of the sciatic nerve.

Sleep hygiene

The conditions and practices promoting continuous and quality sleep. Sleep hygiene includes bedtime routines, regular bed and arise times, as well as, regularly receiving enough sleep to avoid sleepiness during the day.

Soft tissue

The ligaments, tendons and muscles. An acute or chronic overloading of the soft tissue is the most common cause of lower back pain which lies at the basis of nearly 80 percent of back symptoms.

Spinalis

Relating to the spinal column.

Spinal canal

All vertebrae have a 'hole'. 'Stacked' on top of each other, these holes form the spinal canal. Within the spinal canal lies the spinal cord, an important part of the central nervous system. The spinal cord is suspended like a 'tail' from the brain. Nerve roots spring from both sides of the spinal cord and branch outside of the spinal canal onto smaller nerves that run to all parts of the body. The nerve roots leave the spinal canal through openings between the vertebral bodies and the joint protrusions, approximately at the level of the intervertebral disc.

Spinal column segment

Together with the overlying and underlying vertebra, the inter-vertebral disc forms a single segment. Also located within this segment are the facet joints with their joint capsule, all the ligaments between the two vertebrae and the emerging nerves.

Spinal cord

Medulla spinalis; the cord of 31 pairs of nerves which extends from the cerebellum to the first or second lumbar vertebra in the cavity of the spinal column.

Spinal fluid

Fluid in the spinal canal, which is integral with the cerebral fluid in the brain cavities.

Spinal nerves

31 pairs of nerves that emerge from both sides of the spinal cord.

Sacroiliac joint

Joint between the sacrum and the iliac bone (pelvis).

Spinous process
Bony protrusion (processus spinosus) on the vertebra that point almost straight backwards. One can clearly see and feel the spinous processes as a row of vertical bumps in the middle of the back.

Spinal stenosis
Narrowing of the spinal canal.

Stenosis
Narrowing of an opening or canal.

Stimulus
Perceptible change that elicits a response in an organism.

Tailbone
The tailbone (also called coccyx or caudal vertebra) consists (on average) of four bones, which can hardly still be discerned to be vertebrae, and which are fused with the sacrum.

Thermoregulation
The maintenance of the temperature.

Thoracic Outlet Syndrome (TOS)
TOS or shoulder-girdle syndrome is the collective term for disorders in which the neurovascular bundle in the shoulder area has become compressed.

Thorax
Chest.

Tonus
The state of tension in tissues, primarily muscles.

Torticollis
Dystonia; stiff neck coupled with involuntary tension in one or more muscles of the neck, leading to an abnormal position and/or abnormal movements of the head.

Traction
Pulling.

Transverse process
Bony protrusion on the vertebra. Each vertebra has two protruding transverse processes, one pointing to the left and one pointing to the right.

Trauma
Accident, resulting in an injury (both in the physical and mental sense).

Varicose vein
Varix, dilation of veins, primarily in the lower legs because of obstruction in the blood flow (hindrance of the return flow of blood to the heart) and/or vascular wall degeneration.

Vascularisation
Development of blood vessels in an organ or part of organ.

Veins
The blood vessels through which the blood flows back from the body to the heart.

Venous
Relating to the veins.

Venules
Small veins.

Vertebra
Each of the small bones that make up the backbone

Vertebral arch (arcus vertebrae)
On the rear (posterior side) of the vertebra, the vertebral arch can be found. Together with the vertebral body, this forms the spinal canal.

Vertebral body (corpus vertebrae)
The vertebral body is the largest bony part of a vertebra and has the shape of a high, and more or less round disc, which is somewhat flattened at the rear. The vertebral bodies are located on the front side (anterior side) of the spinal column.

Vertebral foramen
Vertebral opening, cavity between the vertebral body and the vertebral arches. The totality of the vertebral foramina forms the spinal canal.

Whiplash
Injury to the neck resulting from an accident or other sudden event in which the head is forcefully moved first backwards and then forwards.

Bibliography

×   Adams, M.A. & P. Dolan (eds.), 'Diurnal changes in spinal mechanics and their clinical significance'. In: *Journal of Bone & Joint Surgery* 72B (1990), nr. 2, pp. 266-270.

×   Adams, M.A. & W.C. Hutton, 'Gradual disc prolapse'. In: *Spine* 10 (1985), nr. 6, pp. 524-531.

×   Adams, M.A. & W.C. Hutton, 'Prolapsed inter-vertebral disc: a hyperflexion injury'. In: *Spine* 7 (1982), nr. 3, pp. 184-191.

×   Adams, M.A. & W.C. Hutton, 'The effect of posture on the lumbar spine'. In: *Journal of Bone & Joint Surgery* 67B (1985), nr. 4.

×   Adams, M.A. & W.C. Hutton, 'The mechanical function of the lumbar apophyseal joints'. In: *Spine* 8 (1983), nr. 3, pp. 327-330.

×   Adams, M.A., W.C. Hutton & J.R. Stott, 'The resistance to flexion of the lumbar inter-vertebral joint'. In: *Spine* 5 (1980), nr. 3, p. 245.

×   Aertgeerts, F., 'Ligkomfort, van plank tot waterbed'. In: *Balanceren op het raakvlak tussen ergonomie en ekologie*, s.l. 1993, pp. 5.1-5.6.

×   Alihanka, J. & K. Vaahtoranta, 'A static charge sensitive bed. A new method for recording body movements during sleep'. In: *Electroencephalography & Clinical Neurophysiology* (1979), nr. 46, pp. 731-734.

×   Allen, V., D.W. Ryan & A. Murray, 'Air-fluidized beds and their ability to disturb interface pressures generated between the subject and the bed surface'. In: *Physiological Measurement* (1993), pp. 359-364.

×   Allen, V., D.W Ryan & A. Murray, 'Potential for bed sores due to high pressures: influence of body sites, body position, and mattress design'. In: *British Journal of Clinical Practice*, 1993 July, Aug; 47 (4): pp. 195-197.

×   Alsaadi S.M., McAuley J.H., Hush J.M., 'Prevalence of sleep disturbance in patients with lower back pain'. In: *European Spine Journal* (2011), 20, pp. 737-743.

×   Ambrogio N., Cuttiford J., Lineker S., Li L., 'A comparison of three types of neck support in fibromyalgia patients'. In: *Arthritis Care Res.*, 1998, vol. 11, nr. 5, pp. 405-410.

×   Anders D., Gompper B., Kräuchi K., 'A two-night comparison in the sleep laboratory as a tool to challenge the relationship between sleep initiation, cardiophysiological and thermoregulatory changes in women with difficulties initiating sleep and thermal discomfort'. In: *Physiol. Behaviour* (2013), 114-115: pp. 77-82.

×   Anderson, M., 'Rückenschule'. In: *Deutsche Krankenpflege Zeitschrift* 46 (1993), nr. 3, pp. 181-186.

×   Andersson, G.B.J. & T.W. McNeill, *Lumbar spine syndromes: evaluation and treatment*, Springer, New York, 1989.

×   Anoniem, Document aan P. Mannekens over slapen en rugklachten. Privé-verzameling Firma ls Bedding, getypt, Maldegem s.a.

×   Anoniem, 'Slaapcomfort: de verschillende onderdelen'. In: Drukkerij Oranje, Sint-Baafs-Vijve, *Meubihome* (1992), nr. 2, pp. 20-30.

×   Anoniem, 'Slaapmiddelen: welke is het minste kwaad?'. In: *Test-Aankoop* (1990), nr. 327, pp. 4-7.

×   Anoniem, *Zo kiest u een goed bed*, Consumentenbond, 1987, pp. 218-222.

×   Artner J., Cakir B., Spiekermann J.A. et al. 'Prevalence of sleep deprivation in patients with chronic neck and back pain: a retrospective evaluation of 1016 patients'. In: *Journal of Pain Research* (2013), 6, pp. 1-6.

×   Atlas S.J., Volinn E., 'Classics from the spine literature revisited: a randomized trial of 2 versus 7 days of recommended bed rest for acute lower back pain'. In: *Spine*, vol. 22, nr. 20, pp. 2331-2337.

×   Bach V., Tellieze F., Libert J.P., 'The interaction between sleep and thermoregulation in adults and neonates'. In: *Sleep Medical Rev.* (2002), nr. 6, (6), pp. 481-492.

×   Bach V., Telliez F., Chardon K., Tourneux P., Cardot V., Libert J.P., 'Thermoregulation in wakefulness and sleep in humans'. In: *Handbook of Clinical Neurology*, vol. 98 (3rd series) Sleep disorders, Part 1, 2011.

×   Bader G.G., Engdal S., 'The influence of bed firmness on sleep quality'. In: *Applied Ergonomics* (2000), 31 (5), pp. 487-497.

×   Bahouq H., Allali F., Rkain H. et al., 'Prevalence and severity of insomnia in chronic lower back pain patients'. In: *Journal of Rheumatology International* (2013), vol. 33, issue 5, pp. 1277-1281.

×   Balagué F., Mannion A.F., et al., *Clinical update: lower back pain*, www.thelancet.com, vol. 369, March 3, 2007.

×   Bartrow K., *Schwachstelle Rücken – Gezielt und effektiv:übungen gegen den Schmerz*, Trias, 2014, Stuttgart

×   Bastiaans, J., 'Psychosomatiek en lage rugklachten'. In: *Nederlands Tijdschrift voor Fysiotherapie* 90 (1980), nr. 3, pp. 106-109.

×   Baumgartner, H., 'Die Bedeuting des Liegekomforts für die Wirbelsäule'. In: *Hospitalis* (1975), nr. 2.

×   Belavy D.L., Bansmann P.M., Böhme G. et al., Changes in inter-vertebral disc morphology persist 5 months after 21-day bed rest'. In: *Journal of Applied Physiology* (2011), vol. 111, pp. 1304-1314.

×   Bell, G.R. & R.H. Rothman, 'The conservative treatment of sciata'. In: *Spine* 9 (1984), nr. 1, pp. 54-56.

×   Bernateck M., Karst M. et al. 'Sustained effects of comprehensive inpatient rehabilitative treatment and sleeping neck support in patients with chronic cervicobrachialgia: a prospective and randomized clinical trial'. In: *International Journal of Rehabilitation Residence* (2008), vol. 31, nr. 4, pp. 342-346.

×   Beunen, G. & R. Renson, *Kinantropometrie en biometrie*. Acco, Leuven, 1988, pp. 104-107.

×   Biedermann, F., 'Über das gesunde Liegen im Bett'. In: *Zeitschrift für Allgemeinmedizin* 50 (1974), nr. 19, pp. 885-887.

×   Biering-Sörensen, F. 'Physical measurements as risk indicators for lower back trouble over a one-year period'. In: *Spine* 9 (1982), nr. 2.

×   Boer, R. de & L.P.S. van der Geest, 'House-dust mite (Pyroglyphidae) populations in mattresses, and their control by electric blankets'. In: *Experimental-Applied Acarology* (1990), nr. 9, pp. 113-122.

×   Bognuk, N., 'Anatomie en functie van de lumbale rugspieren'. In: G.P. Grieve (red.), *Moderne manuele therapie van de wervelkolom* (deel 1), De Tijdstroom, Lochem 1988, pp. 160-166.

×   Boudri, H.C., 'Preventie fysiotherapie en ergonomie'. In: *Nederlands Tijdschrift voor Fysiotherapie* 93 (1983), nr. 5, pp. 153-162.

×   Brands, C. & N. Bergh, 'Adviezen bij aanschaf van een stoel en bed'. Eindexamenscriptie. Hogeschool Eindhoven, studierichting Fysiotherapie, Eindhoven, 1990.

×   Browman, C.P., 'The first-night effect on sleep and dreams'. In: *Biolog. Psychiat.* 15 (1980), pp. 809-812.

×   Bruggeman, A. & J.H. Bruggeman, 'Visuele instructies bij primair discogene aandoeningen van de lumbale wervelkolom'. In: *Nederlands Tijdschrift voor Fysiotherapie* 92 (1982), nr. 12, pp. 318-325.

×   Burgess H.J., Holmes A.L., Dawson D., 'The relationship between slow-wave activity, body temperature, and cardiac activity during nighttime sleep'. In: *Sleep* (2001), vol. 24 (3), pp. 343-349.

×   Burton K., 'How to prevent back pain'. In: *Best Practice & Research Clinical Rheumatology*, (2005), vol. 19, nr. 4, pp. 541-555.

×   Busquet, L., *Les chaines musculaires: tronc et colonne cervicale* (Tome 1). Deuxième édition. Frison-Roche, Paris, 1992.

×   Buckle P., Fernandes A., 'Mattress evaluation, assessment of contact pressure, comfort and discomfort'. In: *Applied Ergonomics* (1998), vol. 29, Issue 1, pp.35-39.

×   Cailliet, R., *Lower back pain syndrome*, 2nd edition, F.A. Davis, Philadelphia, 1976.

×   Cailliet, R., *Neck & arm pain*, 3rd edition, F.A. Davis, Philadelphia, 1991.

×   Cardon G., Geldhof E., Cnockaert B., Janda I., *De Kinderrugschool – Een multifactorieel programma voor een rugvriendelijke levensstijl*, Acco, 2007, Leuven.

×   Carswell, F. & D.W. Robinson (eds.), 'House dust mites in Bristol'. In: *Clin. Allergy* (1982), nr. 12, p. 533.

×   Centrum voor Evaluatie en Revalidatie van Motorische Functies, U.Z. Gasthuisberg, Leuven, 1992.

×   Chadwick, P.R., 'Advising patients on back care'. In: *Physiotherapy* 65 (1979), nr. 9, pp. 277-278.

×   Chang-Yu Hsieh & B.W. Yeung, 'Bed transfer for unilateral sacroiliac pain'. In: *Journal of Orthopaedic & Sports Physical Therapy* (1984), nr. 6, pp. 140-141.

×   Chih-Shan, L. & W. Gwo-Hwa (eds.), 'Seasonal variation of house dust mite allergen (der p I) in a subtropical climate'. In: *J. Allergy Clin. Immunol.* 94 (1994), nr. 1, pp. 131-134.

×   Clark, M. & J. Andreus, 'Comparison of interface pressure measured at the sacrum while resting upon two types of foam mattresses and between platilon and plastic mattress covers'. In: *Age and Ageing* (1991), nr. 20, pp. 267-270.

×   Clarke A., Jones A., O'Malley M., McLaren R., *ABC of Spinal Disorders*, Wiley-Blackwell, UK, 2010.

×   Coëlho, M.B. & G. Kloosterhuis, *Zakwoordenboek der geneeskunde*, 23ste druk, Koninklijke PBNA, Arnhem, 1989.

×   Coenen L., 'De slaap en het bed:een psychobiologische beschouwing' (2006). In: *Medische antropologie*, 18, pp. 133-148.

×   Consumentenbond, *Matrassentest*, oktober 2013.

×   Courtial, D.C., 'The patient with lower back pain: bed positioning'. In: *Hospital Management* 109 (1970), nr. 4, pp. 66-70.

×   Custom8 NV, *Technical Report UC201212-1/ Influence of gel particels on microclimate in latex samples*, 2012.

× Cyriax, J., 'Diagnosis of soft tissue lesions'. In: *Textbook of Orthopaedic Medicine*, vol. 1, 7th edition. Baillière Tindall, London, 1987.

× Cyriax, J., 'Orthopaedic beds'. In: *British Medical Journal* 263 (1975), nr. 5977, p. 231.

× Damms, V.G.S., 'Bed backage'. In: *British Journal of General Practice* 43 (1993), nr. 370, p. 219.

× Davidson J.R., Moldofsky H., Lue F.A., 'Growth hormone and cortisol secretion in relation to sleep and wakefulness'. In: *Journal of Psychiatric Neuroscience* (1991), vol. 16, nr. 2, pp. 96-102.

× Debacker, C., 'Koop geen matras zonder ze te proberen'. In: *Kies keurig* (s.a.), nr. 11, pp. 101-102.

× De Deyne P., 'Application of passive stretch and its implications for muscle fibers'. In: *Physical Therapy* (2001), vol. 81 (2), pp. 819-827.

× Defloot T., 'The effect of position and mattress on interface pressure'. In: *Applied Nursing Research*, vol. 13 (1), (2000), pp. 2-11.

× Delport, H.P. & M.J. Hoogmartens, 'Rugpijn in de auto'. In: *Tijdschrift voor Geneeskunde* 38 (1982), nr. 18, pp. 1173-1175.

× Demotes-Mainard, J., *A quoi bon dormir*, Editions Frison-Roche/Editions espaces 34, Paris, 1992.

× Denne, W., 'An objective assessment of the sheepskin used for decubitus sore prophylaxis'. In: *Rheumatology & Rehabilitation* (1979), nr. 1, pp. 23-29.

× Desantana J.M., Sluka K.A., 'Central mechanisms in the maintenance of chronic widespread non-inflammatory muscle pain'. In: *Curr. Pain Headache report* (2008), 12 (5), pp. 338-343.

× De Vocht J.W., Wilder D.G., Bandstra E.R., Spratt K.F., 'Biomechanical evaluation of four different mattresses'. In: *Applied Ergonomics* (2006), 37, pp. 294-304.

× Dewasmes G., Telliez F., Muzet A., 'Effects of a nocturnal environment perceived as warm on subsequent daytime sleep in humans'. In: *Sleep* (2000), 23 (3), pp. 409-413;

× Deyo, R.A., 'Conservative therapy of lower back pain'. In: *JAMA* (1983), nr. 250: pp. 1057-1062.

× Deyo, R.A., A.K. Diehl & M. Rosenthal, 'How many days of bed rest for acute lower back pain? A randomized clinical trial'. In: *New England Journal of Medicine* (1986), nr. 316, pp. 1064-1070.

× Dickson, P.R., 'Effect of a fleecy woollen underlay on sleep'. In: *Medical Journal of Australia* (1984), nr. 21, pp. 87-89.

× Donatelli, R.A., *Physical therapy of the shoulder*, 2nd edition, Churchill Livingstone, New York 1991.

× Drift, J.H.A. van der, 'Neurologische aspecten van lage rugpijnen'. In: *Nederlands Tijdschrift voor Fysiotherapie* (1980), nr. 3, pp. 202-205.

× Dunn K.M., Campbell P., Jordan K.P., 'Long-term trajectories of back pain: cohort study with 7-year follow-up'. In: *BMJ Open* (2013), 3 (12):e003838.

× Dzvonik, M.L. & D.F. Kripke (eds.), 'Body position changes and periodic movements in sleep'. In: *Sleep* 9 (1986), nr. 4, pp. 484-491.

× Eklundh, M., *Achte auf deinen Rücken!*, 2. Auflage. Pflaum, München, 1979.

× El, A. van der, *Manuele diagnostiek wervelkolom*, Manthel, Rotterdam 1992.

× Elkhuizen J.W., *Stijve rug en nek na verkeerd liggen*, www.ligwijzer.nl

218

×   Enck P., Walten T., Traue H.C., 'Zusammenhänge zwischen Rückenschmerzen, Schlaf und Matratzenqualität, Doppelblinde pilotstudie bei hotelgästen'. In: *Der Schmerz* (1999), 13 (3), pp. 205-207.

×   Ensor J., Oexman R., Scott D., Carrier J., Davis J., *Evaluation of a custom fit solo construction sleep surface using objective and subjective measures of sleep qaulity.* Sleep to Live Institute, 2008, Joplin USA.

×   Erfanian P., Tenzif S., Guerriero R.C., 'Assessing effects of a semi-customized cervical pillow on symptomatic adults with chronic neck pain with and without headache'. In: *The Journal of the Canadian Chiropractic Association*, 2004, vol. 48, nr. 1, pp. 20-28.

×   Ernst, E., 'Lumbago: Ruhe oder Bewegung?'. In: *Fortschr. Med.* 109 (1991), nr. 13, pp. 271-272.

×   Farfan, H.F., *Mechanical disorders of the lower back.* Lea & Febiger, Philadelphia, 1973, pp. 112-113.

×   Farioli A., Mattioli S. et al. ' Musculoskeletal pain in Europe: the role of personal, accupational, and social risk factors'. In: *Scandinavian Journal of Work, environment & health* (2008), vol. 34 (2), pp. 120-132.

×   Fast, A., 'Lower back disorders: conservative management'. In: *Archives of Physical Medicine & Rehabilitation* (1988), nr. 69, pp. 880-891.

×   Folkert, H.F., 'Versuch einer Beweisführung über die günstigste Schlafmöglichkeit bei vertebragenen Schmerzzuständen'. In: *Manuelle Medizin* 9 (1971), nr. 1, pp. 15-18.

×   Frazier, L.M., S.C. Timothy & M.F. Lyles, 'Lengthy bed rest prescribed for acute lower back pain: experience at three general medicine walk-in clinics'. In: *Southern Medical Journal* 84 (1991), nr. 5, pp. 603-606.

×   Frisina, W., 'Study of cradle and pendulum motion for applications to health care'. In: *Journal of Biomechanics* 17 (1984), nr. 8, pp. 573-577.

×   Fronczek R., Raymann R.J.E.M. et al. 'Manipulation of skin temperature improves noctural sleep in narcolepsy'. In: *J. Neurol. Neurosurgery and Psychiatry* (2008), 79, pp. 1354-1357.

×   Fronczek R., Raymann R.J.E.M. et al. 'Manipulation of core body and skin temperature improves vigilance and maintenance of wakefulness in narcolepsy'. In: *Sleep* (2008), 31, pp. 233-240.

×   Frymoyer, J.W., 'Back pain and sciatica'. In: *New England Journal of Medicine* (1988), nr. 318, pp. 291-300.

×   Garfin, S.R. & Pye S.A., 'Bed design and its effect on chronic lower back pain: a limited controlled trial'. In: *Pain* (1981), nr. 10, pp. 87-91.

×   Geus, G. de, 'Biomechanische achtergronden van de laag lumbale discusproblematiek'. In: *Nederlands Tijdschrift voor Fysiotherapie* 92 (1982), nr. 2, pp. 24-27.

×   Gemeenschappelijke Medische Dienst (gmd), *Elektrisch verstelbare hoog-laagbedden voor de thuissituatie. Deel 3: definities en meetprocedures.* Amsterdam 1990.

×   Goel, V.K., 'The role of lumbar spinal elements in flexion'. In: *Spine* 10 (1985), nr. 6, pp. 516-523.

×   Gogia, P.P., 'Bed rest effect on extremity muscle torque in healthy men'. In: *Archives of Physical Medicine & Rehabilitation* (1989), nr. 69, pp. 1030-1032.

×   Goossens, R.H.M. & C.J. Snijders (eds.), 'A new instrument for measurement of forces on beds and seats'. In: *J. Biomed. Eng.* (1993), nr. 15, pp. 409-412.

×   Gordon S.J., Grimmer-Somers K., Trott P., 'Pillow use: the behaviour of cervical pain, sleep quality and pillow comfort in side sleepers'. In: *Manual Therapy* (2009), vol. 14, nr. 6, pp. 671-680.

×   Gordon S.J., Grimmer-Somers K.A., Trott P.H., 'Pillow use: the behavior of cervical stiffness, headache and scapular/arm pain'. In: *Journal of Pain Research* (2010), vol. 11, nr. 3, pp. 137-145.

×   Gottschalk, E., 'Das "Brett im Bett" genügt noch nicht'. In: *Der Landarzt* (1966), nr. 34, pp. 1534-1536.

×   Gravovetsky, S.A., 'The resting spine: a conceptual approach to the avoidance of spinal reinjury during rest'. In: *Physical Therapy* 67 (1987), nr. 4, pp. 549-553.

×   Grieve, G.P., *De wervelkolom*, De Tijdstroom, Lochem 1991.

×   Grubb, S.A. et al., 'The relative value of lumbar roentgenograms, metrizamide myelography and discography in the assessment of patients with chronic low-back syndrome'. In: *Spine* 12 (1987), nr. 3, pp. 282-286.

×   Günter, D., 'Die ideale Liege: elastisch und fest zugleich'. In: *Möbel Cultur* (1977), nr. 10, pp. 146-152.

×   Guttmann, L., 'The prevention and treatment of pressure sores'. In: *Bedsore biomechanics: Proceedings of a seminar on tissue viability*, University of Strathclyde, Glasgow 1975.

×   Gwendolen, A.J., 'De behandeling van acute lage rugpijn'. In: G.P. Grieve (red), *Moderne manuele therapie van de wervelkolom* (deel 2), De Tijdstroom, Lochem 1989, pp. 786-793.

×   Gwendolen, A.J., 'Onderzoek van de lendewervelkolom'. In: G.P. Grieve (red.), *Moderne manuele therapie van de wervelkolom* (deel 2), De Tijdstroom, Lochem 1989, pp. 586-598.

×   Haarlemmer A.F., Soerjanto R., Fibromyalgie, *Inleiding voor artsen, patiënten en arbeidskundigen*, De Tijdstroom, 1996, Utrecht.

×   Hadler N.M., Evans A.T., 'Medium-firm mattresses reduced pain-related disability more than firm mattress in chronic, non-specific low-back pain'. In: *ACP J Club* (2004), 141, 12.

×   Haex B., *Back and Bed: Ergonomic Aspects of Sleeping*. Boca Raton, CRC Press, 2005.

×   Hagen K.B., Hilde G., Jamtveldt G., Winnem M.F., 'The Cochrane review of bed rest for acute lower back pain and sciatica'. In: *Spine* (2000), vol. 25, nr. 22, pp. 2932-2939.

×   Hagen K.B., Hilde G., Jamtveldt G., Winnem M.F., 'The Cochrane review of advice to stay active as a single treatment for lower back pain and sciatica', In: *Spine* (2002), vol. 27, nr. 16, pp. 1736-1741.

×   Hagen K.B., Hilde G., Jamtveldt G., Winnem M., 'Bed rest for acute low-back pain and sciatica'. In: *Cochrane Database Systematic Review*. (2004), (4), CD001254.

×   Hagen KB., Jamtveldt G., Hilde G., Winnem M.F., 'The updated Cochrane review of bed rest for lower back pain and sciatica'. In: *Spine* (2005), 30 (5), pp. 542-546.

×   Hagino C, Erfanian P., 'Before/after study to determine the effectiveness of an adjustable wood frame, foam and wool mattress bed-system in reducing chronic back pain in adults'. In: *Journal of Canadian Chriropractic Association* (1997), (41), pp. 16-26.

×   Hagino C., Boscariol J., Dover L., Letendre R., Wicks M., 'Before/after study to determine the effectiveness of the align-right cylindrical cervical pillow in reducing chronic neck pain severity'. In: *Journal of Manipulative and Physiological Therapeutics*, 1998; vol. 21, nr. 2, pp. 89-93.

×   Harman K., Pivik R.T., D'Eon J.L., Wilson K.G., Swenson J.R., Matsunaga L., 'Sleep in depressed and non-depressed participants with chronic lower back pain: electroencephalographic and behavior findings'. In: *Sleep* (2002), vol. 25, pp. 775-783.

×   Haskell, E.H. & J.W. Palca, 'The influence of ambient temperatures on electrophysiological sleep in humans'. In: *Sleep Research* (1978), nr. 7, pp. 169-170.

×   Hauri, P., *The sleep disorders: current concepts*, Upjohn Company, Michigan, 1977.

×   Hauri, P. & D.R. Hawkins, 'Alpha-delta sleep'. In: *Electroencephalography Clin. Neurophysiol.* (1973), nr. 34, pp. 233-237.

×   Hauri, P. & S. Linde, *No more sleepless nights*, John Wiley & Sons, New York 1990.

×   Hearn, E. ,*You are as young as your spine. Heinemann*, W.M.B. (ed.), Ackford R.J., Great Britain 1975.

×   Heidinger F., 'Ergonomic functional testing of the biomechanical properties of the latex-mattress 'Ergo Pro Innergetic' with different cover versions', Test Report ELK/30/2013, In: *Ergonomie, Institut München* (2013), pp.1-27.

×   Heidinger F. 'Ergonomische Untersuchungen zu den biomechanischen und mikroklimatischen eigenschaften von latex- und taschenfederkern-matratzen in verbindung mit boxspring-unterfederungen, Untersuchungsbericht'. In: *Ergonomie Institut München* (2007), pp. 1-20.

×   Heijden, G.J.M.G. van der & L.M. Bouter (eds.), 'Effectiviteit van tractie bij lage rugklachten'. In: *Nederlands Tijdschrift voor Fysiotherapie* 100 (1990), nr. 6, pp. 163-167.

×   Helewa A., Goldsmith C.H., Smythe H.A., Lee P., Obright K., Stitt L., 'Effect of therapeutic exercise and sleeping neck support on patients with chronic neck pain: a randomized clinical trial'. In: *Journal of Rheumatology*, 2007, vol. 34, nr. 1, pp. 151-158.

×   Henane R., Buguet A., Roussel B., Bittel J., 'Variations in evaporation and body temperatures during sleep in man;. In: *Journal of Applied Physiology* (1977), vol. 42 (1), pp. 50-55.

×   Hijdra A., Koudstaal P.J., Roos R.A.C., *Neurologie*, 3e druk, Elsevier Gezondheidszorg, Maarssen, 2003.

×   Hill, H., 'Backache relieved by polystyrene mattress'. In: *Lancet* (1973), nr. 793, p. 36.

×   Hobson, J.A., T. Spagna & R. Malenka, 'Ethology of sleep studied with time-lapse photography: postural immobility and sleep-cycle phase in humans'. In: *Science* 201 (1978), nr. 29, pp. 1251-1253.

×   Hoddes, E. & V. Zarcone (eds.), 'Quantification of sleepiness: a new approach'. In: *Psychophysiology* (1973), nr. 10, pp. 431-434.

×   Hoekstra, G.R., 'Patiënten met lage rugklachten in een huisartspraktijk'. In: *De Nederlandse bibliotheek der geneeskunde*, deel 181, jaargang 18. Stafleu, s.l. 1983, p. 273.

×   Hofman, A. & R.H. Geelkerken (ed.), 'Pressure sores and pressure-decreasing mattresses: controlled clinical trial'. In: *Lancet* 343 (1994), nr. 8897, pp. 568-571.

×   Hoogmartens, M., 'Rughygiëne: de optimale matrasdikte'. *Tijdschrift voor Geneeskunde* 40 (1984), nr. 11, pp. 699-701.

×   Höppe, P., 'Optimale Schlafbedingungen'. In: *Deutsche Medizinische Wochenschrift* (1991), nr. 2, p. 874.

×   Hoy D., March L., Blyth F. et al., 'The global burden of lower back pain: estimates from the global burden disease 2010 study', In: *Annals Rheumat. Dis.* (2014).

×   Hsieh, C.Y. & Bradley W.Y., 'Bed transfer for unilateral sacroiliac pain'. In: *Journal of Orthopaedic & Sports Physical Therapy* (1984), nr. 6, pp. 140-141.

×   Hurley et al. 'Physiotherapy for sleep disturbance in chronic lower back pain: a feasibility randomized controlled trial'. *BMC Musculoskeletal disorders* (2010) 11, pp. 1-11.

×   Hutton WC., Malko J.A., Fajman W.A., 'Lumbar disc volume measured by MRI: effects of bed rest, horizontal exercise, and vertical loading'. In: *Aviation Space Environ med.*, (2003), 74(1), pp. 73-78.

×   Huysmans T., Haex B., De Wilde T. et al., 'A 3D active shape model for the evaluation of the alignment of the spine during sleep'. *Gait&Posture*, 2004, 24, pp. 54-61.

×   Hyppa, M.T. & E. Kronholm, 'Sleep movements and poor sleep in patients with non-specific somatic complaints: affective disorders and sleep quality'. In: *Journal of Psychosomatic Research* 31 (1987), nr. 5, pp. 631-637.

×   Jacobson B.H.,Gemmell H.A., Hayes B.M., Altena T.S., 'Effectiveness of selected bedding system on quality of sleep, back pain, shoulder pain, and spine stiffness.', In: *Journal of Manipulative and Physiological Therapeutics* (2002), 25(2), pp. 88-92.

×   Jacobson B.H., Wallace T., Gemmell H., 'Subjective rating of perceived back pain, stiffness and sleep quality following introduction of medium-firm bedding systems'. In: *Journal of Chiropractic Medicine* (2006), vol. 5, nr. 4, pp. 128-134.

×   Jacobson BH., Wallace TJ., Smith DB., Kolb T., 'Grouped comparisons of sleep quality for new and personal bedding systems'. In: *Applied Ergonomics* (2008), 39 (2), pp. 247-254.

×   Jacobson B.H., Boolani A., Doug B.S., 'Changes in back pain, sleep quality, and perceived stress after introduction of new bedding systems'. In: *Journal of Chiropractic Medicine* (2009), 8 (1), pp. 1-8.

×   Jacobson B.H., Boolani A., Dunklee G. et al. 'Effect of prescribed sleep surfaces on back pain and sleep quality in patients diagnosed with lower back and shoulder pain'. In: *Applied Ergonomics* (2010), vol. 42(1), pp. 91-97.

×   Jensen, G.M., 'Biomechanics of the lumbar inter-vertebral disc: a review'. In: *Physical Therapy* 60 (1980), nr. 6.

×   Jobe, F.W. & Moynes R.D., 'Delineation of diagnostic criteria and rehabilitation program for rotator cuff injuries'. In: *American Journal Sports Medicine* (1982), nr. 10, p. 366.

×   Jonker, A., 'Decubitus'. In: *Tijdschrift voor Bejaarden-, Kraam- en Ziekenverzorging* (1978), nr. 1, pp. 23-29.

×   Joosten, T., *Bedden*. Eindexamenscriptie. Academie voor Fysiotherapie, Arnhem 1984.

×   Junghanns, H., *Die gesunde und die kranke Wirbelsäule in Röntgenbild und Klinik*. Georg Thieme Verlag, Stuttgart 1968.

×   Jürgens, H.W., *Die Eigenschaften einer guten Matratze und ihre Prüfungsmöglichkeiten*. (10 p.) J. Balteman, privé-verzameling idc, Kiel. s.a.

×   Jürgens H.W., Hausstaubmilben und Bett'.,In: *Der Kinderarzt* (1992), 23, pp. 1884-1889.

×   Kahle, W., H. Leonhardt & W. Platzer, *Sesam atlas van de anatomie* (deel 3). Bosch en Keuning, Baarn, 1991.

×   Kahmann, L.R.M., *Anti-decubitus-ligondersteuningen. Deelproject: Stand van zaken onderzoek ligondersteuningen*. Gemeenschappelijke Medische Dienst, Amsterdam augustus 1991.

×   Kapandji, I.A., *Bewegingsleer. Deel 3: de romp en de wervelkolom*. Bohn, Scheltema & Holkema, Utrecht, 1986.

×   Kawabata A., Tokura H., 'Effects of two kinds of pillow on thermoregulatory responses during night sleep' In: *Applied Human science – Journal of Physiological Anthropology* (1996), vol. 15 (4), pp. 155-159.

×   Kazarian, L.E., 'Creep characteristics of the human spinal column'. In: *Orthop. Clin. North Am.* (1975), nr. 6, pp. 3-18.

×   Keegan, J.J., 'Alternations of the lumbar curve to posture and seating'. In: *Journal of Bone & Joint Surgery* (1951), nr. 35, pp. 589-603.

×   Keim, H.A., 'Scoliosis'. In: *Clinical Symposia* 24 (1972), nr. 1, pp. 13-23.

×   Keim, H.A. & W.H. Kirkaldy-Willis, 'Lower back pain'. In: *Clinical Symposia* (1988), nr. 2.

×   Keller TS., Nathan M., 'Height change caused by creep in inter-vertebral discs: a sagittal plane model'. (1999), *J Spinal Disord*, vol.12, nr. 4, pp. 313-324.

×   Kelly G.A., Blake C., Power C.K., O'Keeffe D., Fullen B.M., 'The association between chronic lower back pain and sleep: a systematic review'. In: *Clinical Journal of Pain* (2011), 27 (2), pp.169-181.

×   Kempf B., Kongsted A., 'Association between the side of unilateral shoulder pain and preferred sleeping position: a cross-sectional study of 83 Danish patients'. In: *Journal of Manipulative Physiological Therapy* (2012), vol. 35, nr. 5, pp. 407-412.

×   Kendall, H.O., F.P. Kendall & D.A. Boynton, *Posture and pain*. The Williams & Wilkins Company, Baltimore 1952.

×   Kendall, F.P. & E.K. McCreary, *Spierfunctie in relatie tot de houding*, Bohn, Scheltema & Holkema, Utrecht 1985.

×   Kendel, K. & W. Schmidt-Kessen, 'The influence of room temperature on night-sleep in man'. In: WP. Koella & P. Levis (eds.), *Sleep*, s.l. 1973, pp. 423-425.

×   Keurmerkinstituut, Brochure over het bed aan P. Mannekens. Voorburg 13/4/1993.

×   Key S., Roberts V., *The back sufferers' pocket guide*, Vermilion, London, 2010.

×   Kingma, M.J. & H.J. Dokta, *Rugpijn*. Bohn, Scheltema & Holkema, Utrecht 1985.

×   Kinkel, H.J. & H. Maxion, 'Schlafphysiologische Untersuchungen zur Beürteilung Verscheidener Matratzen'. In: *Internationale Zeitschrift für angewandte Physiologie* (1970), nr. 28, pp. 247-262.

×   Kirch, K.M., *Slaapstoornissen, natuurlijk behandelen*, Zuidnederlandse Uitgeverij, Aartselaar 1993.

×   Kirkaldy-Willis, E.S.H., 'The back school'. In: W.H. Kirkaldy-Willis (ed.), *Managing lower back pain*, 2nd edition. Churchill Livingstone, New York 1988, pp. 265-285.

×   Kirkaldy-Willis, W.H., 'The mediation of pain'. In: W.H. Kirkaldy-Willis (ed.), *Managing lower back pain*, 2nd edition. Churchill Livingstone, New York 1988, pp. 78-81.

×   Kline, M.V., P.A. Sullivan & L.L. Coleman, 'Some clinical sleep parameters with the innerspace flotation bed: a preliminary report with reference to insomnia'. In: *Journal of the American Society of Psychosomatic Dentistry & Medicine* 21 (1974), nr. 1, pp. 3-9.

×   Knibbe, N.E. & A. van Zuilekom, 'Eigen schuld? U bent snel weer beter...?'. In: *Nederlands Tijdschrift voor Fysiotherapie* 100 (1990), nr. 4, pp. 111-115.

×   Kolen, P. van & P. van Der Wee, *Mijn rug levenslang*. Coda, Antwerpen 1992.

×   Koppert, G., 'Van houten krib tot stalen bedspiraal'. In: *Nederlands Militair Geneeskundig Tijdschrift* 18 (1965), nr. 9, pp. 284-287.

×   Korkala, D., 'Immunohistochemical demonstration of nociceptors in the ligamentous structures of the lumbar spine'. In: *Spine* 9 (1984), nr. 2, pp. 156-158.

×   Korsgaard, J., 'House dust mites and absolute indoor humidity'. In: *Allergy* (1983a), nr. 38, pp. 85-92.

×   Korsgaard, J., 'Preventive measures in mite asthma: a controlled trial'. In: *Allergy* (1983b), nr. 38, pp. 93-94.

×   Kovacs FM., Abraira V., Pena A., Martin-Rodriguez J.G., Sanchez-Vera M., Ferrer E. et al., 'Effect of firmness of mattress on chronic non-specific low-back pain: randomized, double-blind, controlled, multicentre trial'. In: *Lancet* (2003), 15, pp. 1599-1604.

×   Krag, M.H. & Cohen M.C., 'Body height chance during upright and recumbent posture'. In: *Spine* 15 (1990), nr. 3, pp. 202-207.

×   Krahé, L.J., *Reactie op de rugschool*, s.l, 1992, pp. 11-12.

×   Krämer, J., 'Therapie bij lumbale discusprolaps'. In: *Nederlands Tijdschrift voor Fysiotherapie* 100 (1990), nr. 2, pp. 42-47.

×   Kräuchi K., Wirz-Justice A., 'Circadian rhythm of heat production, heart rate, and skin and core temperature under unmasking conditions in men'. In: *The American Journal of Physiology* (1994), 267 (3pt. 2), pp. 819-829.

× Kräuchi K., Cajochen C., Wirz-Justice A., 'A relationship between heat loss and sleepiness: effects of postural change and melatonin administration'. In: *Journal of Applied Physiology* (1997), vol. 83 (1), pp. 134-139.

× Kräuchi K., Deboer T., 'The interrelationship between sleep regulation and thermoregulation'. In: *Front. Bioscience* (2010), vol. 15, pp. 604-625.

× Kuijer, P. & B. Visser, 'Ergonomische aspecten van het zitten'. In: *Nederlands Tijdschrift voor Fysiotherapie* 102 (1992), nr. 2, pp. 34-37.

× Kushner, I., A. Forer & A.B. McGuire, *Understanding arthritis*, Consumers Union, Mount Vernon 1985, pp. 40-41.

× Kusunoki, M., 'Body movements during sleep as an indicator of comfort'. In: *Japanese Journal of Hygiene* 39 (1985), nr. 6, pp. 886-893.

× La Ban, M.M., '"Vespers curse" night pain: the bane of Hypnos'. In: *Archives of Physical Medicine & Rehabilitation* (1984), nr. 9, pp. 501-504.

× Lahm R., Iaizzo P.A., 'Physiologic responses during rest on a sleep system at varied degrees of firmness in a normal population'. In: *Ergonomics* (2002), vol. 45, nr. 11, pp. 798-815.

× Landesgewerbeanstalt Bayern, Afschrift van 'Industrieantropologische Prüfung' aan P. Coninck, Nürnberg. Privé-verzameling P. Coninck, Brussel, getypt, s.a., pp. 27-44.

× Lavin R.A, Pappagallo M., Kuhlenmeier K.V., 'Cervical Pain: a comparison of three pillows'. In: *Arch. Phys. Med. Rehabilitation* (1997), (78), pp. 193-198.

× Lavigne G.S, Velly-Miguel A.M, Montplaisier J., 'Muscle pain, dyskinesia, and sleep.' In: *Canadian Journal of Physiological Pharmacology* (1991), 61, pp. 678-682.

× Lee, C.K., 'Office management of lower back pain'. In: *Ortho. Clin. North Am.* (1988), nr. 19, pp. 797-804.

× Lee J.H., Choi H.S., Yang S.N., et al., 'True neurogenic thoracic outlet syndrome following hyperabduction during sleep- a case report'. In: *Annals of Rehabilitation Medicine* (2011) vol.35, nr. 4, p. 565-569.

× Leigh, T.J. & I. Hindmarch (eds.), 'Comparison of sleep in osteoarthritic patients and age and sex matched healthy controls'. In: *Annals of the Rheumatic Diseases* (1988), nr. 47, pp. 40-42.

× Leifeld U., Wieland C., *Himmlisch schlafen – Ein Ratgeber rund um gesunden Schlaf*. Oldib, 2010, Essen.

× Leilnahari K. et al., 'Spine aligment in men during lateral sleep position:experimental study and modeling'. In: *BioMedical Engineering OnLine* (2011), 10:103.

× Leroy, B. & M. van Tongele, *De gedroomde slaap: medisch advies voor een betere slaap*. Lannoo (Tielt), 1995.

× Levy H., Hutton W.C., 'Mattresses and sleep for patients with lower back pain: a survey of orthopaedic surgeons'. In: *Journal of South Orthopedic Association* (1996), 5, pp. 185-187.

× Libert J.P., La regulation thermique au cours du sommeil'. In: *Revue Neurologique* (2003), vol. 159 nr. 11, 6S30-4.

× Lilla, J., R. Friedrichs & L. Vistnes, 'Flotation mattress for prevention and treatment of tissue breakdown'. In: *Geriatrics* (1975), nr. 9, pp. 71-75.

× Li-Ping W., Yi-Kai L. et al., 'Morphological changes of the in vitro cervical vertebral canal and its cast form during flexion, extension, and lateral bending'. In: *Journal of Manipulative and Physiological Therapeutics* (2010), pp. 132-137.

× Lorrain, D., J. De Koninck, H. Dionne & G. Goupil, 'Sleep positions and postural shifts in elderly persons'. In: *Perceptual & Motor Skills* (1986), nr. 63, pp. 352-354.

× Maesschalck, V., *Slapen en rugklachten*, Eindwerk. Hoger Instituut Coloma voor kinesitherapie, Mechelen 1995.

×   MacNab, I., Backache, Williams & Wilkins Co., *Back Pain in an Adolescent-Reply*, Baltimore 1977.

×   Magarey, M.E., 'De eerste zitting van de behandeling'. In: G.P. Grieve (ed.), *Moderne manuele therapie van de wervelkolom* (deel 2), De Tijdstroom, Lochem 1989, pp. 702-711.

×   Mahakittikun V., Jirapongsananuruk O. et al., 'Woven material for bed encasement prevents mite penetration'. In: *Journal of Allergy and Clinical Immunology* (2003), vol. 112(6), pp. 1239-1241.

×   Maklebust, J.A., 'Pressure ulcers: etiology and prevention'. In: *Nurs. Clin. North. Am.* 22 (1987), nr. 2, pp. 359-377.

×   Malko J.A., Hutton W.C., Fajman W.A., 'An in vivo MRI study of the changes in volume (and fluid content) of the lumbar inter-vertebral disc after overnight bed rest and during an 8-hour walking protocol'. In: *Journal of Spinal Disorders Tech.*, (2002), 15(2), pp. 157-163.

×   Malcolm, I.V.J., *The lumbar spine and back pain*, 4th edition. Churchill Livingstone, New York 1992.

×   Malmivaara A., Hakkinen U., Aro T. et al., 'The treatment of acute lower back pain — bed rest, exercises or ordinary activity?'. In: *New England Journal of Medicine*, 1995: 332: pp. 351-355.

×   Mannekens, P., *Radiologische evaluatie van drie verschillende slaapsystemen ter preventie van rugklachten*. Licentiaatsverhandeling motorische revalidatie en kinesitherapie, Katholieke Universiteit Leuven, Leuven 1993.

×   Mannekens, P., *Rug en Bed. Slaapsystemen en de preventie van rugklachten*, Elsevier/De Tijdstroom, Maarsen 1997.

×   Marchand, F. & A.M. Ahmed, 'Investigation of the laminate structure of lumbar disc anulus fibrosus'. In: *Spine* 14 (1989), nr. 2, pp. 166-167.

×   Marty M., Rozenberg S., Duplan B., Thomas P., Duquesnoy B., Allaert F., 'Quality of sleep in patients with chronic lower back pain: a case-control study'. In: *European Spine Journal* (200), 17, pp. 839-844.,

×   Maruta, T. & D. Osborne, 'Sexual activity in chronic pain patients'. In: *Psychosomatics* 19 (1978), nr. 9, pp. 531-537.

×   Massey, A.E., 'De bewegingen van voor pijn gevoelige structuren in het wervelkanaal', In: G.P. Grieve (ed.), *Moderne manuele therapie van de wervelkolom* (deel 1), De Tijdstroom, Lochem, 1988, pp. 206-216.

×   Matsumura Y., Kasai Y., Obata H., Matsushima S., Inaba T., Uchida A., 'Changes in water content of inter-vertebral discs and paravertebral muscles before and after bed rest'. In: *Journal of Orthopedic Science* (2009), 14 (1), pp. 45-50.

×   Matthews, M., 'De fysiotherapeutische behandeling van de "whiplash"-patiënt'". In: G.P. Grieve (ed.), *Moderne manuele therapie van de wervelkolom* (deel 2), De Tijdstroom, Lochem 1989.

×   McKenzie, R., *Treat your own neck*. Spinal publications, New Zealand 1983.

×   McKenzie R., *Treat your own back*, 4th edition. Spinal publications, New Zealand 1988.

×   Meerwijk, G.M. van, 'De patiënt na H.N.P. operatie: stabilisatie, mobilisatie en A.D.L.'. In: *Nederlands Tijdschrift voor Fysiotherapie* 94 (1984), nr. 10, pp. 211-216.

×   Meeusen, R. & P. Geerts, *Rugklachten, doe er wat aan!* Lexico België, Kalmthout 1993.

×   Meilach, D.Z., *Rugklachten: voorkomen – genezen*. De Centaur, Amsterdam 1981.

×   Miedema H.S., Van der Molen H.F., Kuijer P.P., Koes B.W., Burdorf A., 'Incidence of lower back pain related occupational diseases in the Netherlands'. In: *European Journal of Pain*, (2013).

× Moffet-Klaber, J.A. 'A controlled, prospective study to evaluate the effectiveness of a lower back school in the relief of chronic lower back pain'. In: *Spine* 11 (1986), nr. 1, pp. 120-122.

× Miller, W.C. (ed.), 'Treatment of insomniac patients with the air-fluidized bed'. In: *American Journal of Psychiatry* 128 (1972), nr. 9, pp. 1147-1150.

× Miranda H., Viikari-Juntura E., Punnett L., Riihimäki H., 'Occupational loading, health behavior and sleep disturbance as predictors of low-back pain'. In: *Scandinavian Journal of Work, Environment & Health*, (2008), vol. 34, nr. 6, p. 411-419.

× Moldofsky, H., 'Sleep and fibrositis syndrome'. In: *Rheumatic Disease Clinics of North America* 15 (1989), nr. 1, pp. 91-103.

× Moldofsky, H., 'Sleep and musculoskeletal pain'. In: *American Journal of Medicine* (1986), nr. 81, suppl.3A, pp. 85-89.

× Moldofsky, H. & F.A. Lue, (eds.), 'Alpha eeg sleep and morning symptoms in rheumatoid arthritis'. In: *Journal of Rheumatology* 10 (1983), nr. 3, pp. 373-379.

× Moldofsky, H. & F.A. Lue (eds.), 'Sleep and morning pain in primary arthrosis'. In: *Journal of Rheumatology* 14 (1987), nr. 1, pp. 124-128.

× Moldofsky, H., P. Scarisbrick, R. England & H. Smythe, 'Musculoskeletal symptoms and non-REM sleep disturbance in patients with "fibrositis syndrome" and healthy subjects'. In: *Psychosomatic Med.* (1975), nr. 37, pp. 341-351.

× Molendijk, M. & I. Colard, 'Drukpunten bij het fibromyalgiesyndroom: de betrouwbaarheid in de dagelijkse praktijk'. In: *Nederlands Tijdschrift voor Fysiotherapie* 101 (1991), nr. 2, pp. 31-36.

× Molony, R.R. & D.M. MacPeek (eds.), 'Sleep, sleep apnea and the fibromyalgia syndrome'. In: *Journal of Rheumatology* 13 (1986), nr. 4, pp. 797-800.

× Monroe, L., 'Psychological and physiological differences between good and poor sleepers'. In: *Journal of Abnormal Psychology* (1967), nr. 72, pp. 255-264.

× Monsein M, Corbin T.P., Culliton P.D., Merz D., Schuck E.A., 'Short-term outcomes of chronic back pain patients on an airbed versus innerspring mattresses'. In: *Medscape General Medicine* (2000), 11;2(3): E36.

× Mooney, V., 'Where is the pain coming from?'. In: *Spine* 12 (1987), nr. 8, pp. 754-759.

× Morree J.J. de, *Dynamiek van het menselijk bindweefsel: functie, beschadiging en herstel*. 2e druk. Bohn Stafleu Van Loghum, Houten, 1993.

× Mosbech, H., A. Jensen, J.H. Heinig & C. Schou, 'House dust mite allergens on different types of mattresses'. In: *Clin. Exp. Allergy* 21 (1991), nr. 3, pp. 351-355.

× Mosbech, H., J. Korsgaard & P. Lind, 'Control of house dust mites by electrical heating blankets'. In: *J Allergy Clin Immunol* 81-ii (1988), nr. 4, pp. 706-710.

× Mosbech, H. & P. Lind, 'Collection of house dust for analysis of mite allergens'. In: *Allergy* (1986), nr. 41, p. 373.

× Moses, J., A. Lubin, P. Naitoh & C. Johnson, 'Reliability of sleep maesures'. In: *Psychophysiology* 9 (1972), nr. 1, pp. 78-82.

× Mueller, R., 'Bandscheiben und bett'. In: *Agnes Karll-Schwester. Der krankpfleger* 21 (1967), nr. 9, pp. 365-366.

× Munir A.K., Einarsson R., Dreborg S.K., 'Vacuum cleaning decreases the levels of mite allergens in house dust'. In: *Pediatric Allergy Immunology*, (1993), 4 (3), pp. 136-143.

× Munoz-Munoz S., Munoz-Garcia M.T. et al., 'Myofascial trigger points, pain, disability, and sleep quality in individuals with mechanical neck pain'. In: *Journal of Manipulative Physiological Therapy* (2012), vol. 35, nr. 8, pp. 608-613.

× Murrie V.L., Wilson H., Hollingworth W., Antoun N.M., Dixon A.K., 'Supportive cushions produce no practical reduction in lumbar lordosis.'. In: *The British Journal of Radiology* (2002), 75, pp. 536-538.

× Muzet, A. & J. Ehrhart, (eds.), 'REM sleep and ambient temperature in man'. In: *International Journal of Neuroscience* (1983), nr. 18, pp. 117-126.

× Nachemson, A.L., 'Recent advances in the treatment of lower back pain'. In: *International Orthopaedics* (1985), nr. 9, pp. 1-10.

× Nachemson, A.L., 'The influence of spinal movements on the lumbar intradiscal pressure and on the tensile stresses in the annulus fibrosus'. In: *Acta Orthopaedica Scandinavica* (1963), nr. 33, pp. 183-207.

× Nachemson, A.L., 'The load on lumbar disc in different positions of the body'. In: *Clinical Orthopaedics & Related Research* (1966), nr. 45, pp. 107-122.

× Nachemson, A.L., 'The lumbar spine: an orthopedic challenge'. In: *Spine* 1 (1976), nr. 1, pp. 59-71.

× Nachemson, A.L., 'Work for all: for those with lower back pain as well'. In: *Clinical Orthopaedics & Related Research* (1983), nr. 179, pp. 77-85.

× Nadler S.F., Steiner D.J. et al., 'Overnight use of continuous low-level heatwrap therapy for relief of lower back pain'. In: *Arch. Physio. Med. Rehabilitation* (2003), vol. 84 (3), pp. 335-342.

× Nakamura M., Nishiwaki Y., Ushida T., Toyama Y., 'Prevalence and characteristics of chronic musculoskeletal pain in Japan: A second survey of people with or without chronic pain'. In: *Journal of Orthopedic Science* (2014) 19, pp. 339-350.

× Nayer, J. de & Y. Xhardez, 'Literie et maux de dos'. In: *Kiné Plus* (1993), nr. 38, pp. 4-12.

× Nederlandse Vereniging van Rubberfabrikanten, *De bekende en onbekende wereld van de zachte 'polyurethaanschuimen'.* S.l., 1983.

× Neumeyer, G., Brief aan W. Vanryckeghem, Hamburg 15-7-1988. Privé-verzameling P. Coninck, Brussel, getypt.

× Nicholson, A.N. & B.M. Stone, 'Influence of back angle on the quality of sleep in seats'. In: *Ergonomics* 30 (1987), nr. 7, pp. 1033-1041.

× Nicol, K. & D. Rusteberg, 'Pressure distribution on mattresses'. In: *Journal of Biomechanics* 26 (1993), nr. 12, pp. 1479-1486.

× Normand M.C., Descarreaux M., Poulin C. et al., 'Biomechanical effects of a lumbar support in a mattress'. In: *Journal of Canadian Chiropractic Association* (2005), 49 (2), p. 96-101.

× O'Donoghue G.M., Fox N., Heneghan C., Hurley D.A., 'Objective and subjective assessment of sleep in chronic lower back pain patients compared with healthy age and gender matched controls: a pilot study'. In: *BioMed Central Musculoskeletal Disorders* (2009), 10, pp. 1-9.

× Oerlemans, H.M., 'Fysiotherapie na een lumbale laminectomie'. In: *Nederlands Tijdschrift voor Fysiotherapie* 98 (1988), nr. 11, pp. 245-251.

× Ogawa, T., T. Satoh & K. Takagi, 'Sweating during night sleep'. In: *Japanese Journal of Physiology* (1967), nr. 17, pp. 135-148.

× Okada, M., M. Chih-Shan & H. Tokura, 'The effects of two different kinds of quilt on human core temperature during night sleep'. In: *Ergonomics* 37 (1994), nr. 5, pp. 851-857.

× Okada S., Suzuki S., Fukui T. et al., *Basic study for optimal control of in-bed temperature during sleep* (2005), Conf. Proc. IEEE Eng. Med. Biol. Soc. (4) pp. 4083-4086.

× Okamoto K, Lizuka S, Okudaira N., 'The effects of air mattress upon sleep and bed climate'. In: *Applied Human Science*, 1997 May, 16(3), pp. 97-102.

×   Okamoto K, Mizuno K, Okudaira N, 'The effects of a newly designed air mattress upon sleep and bed climate'. In: *Applied Human Science*, 1997 July, 16 (4), pp. 161-166.

×   Okamoto-Mizuno K., Michie S., Maeda A., Lizuka S., 'Effects of humid heat exposure on human sleep stages and body temperature'. In: *Sleep* (1999), 22 (6), pp. 767-773.

×   Okamoto-Mizuno K., Tsuzuki K., Mizuno K., 'Effects of mild heat exposure on sleep stages and body temperature in older men'. In: *International Journal of Biometeorology* (2004), 49 (1), pp. 32-36.

×   Okamoto-Mizuno K., Tsuzuki K., Mizuno K., 'Effects of humid heat exposure in later sleep segments on sleep stages and body temperature in humans'. In: *Int. Journal of Biometeorology* (2005), vol. 49 (4), pp. 232-237.

×   Okamoto-Mizuno K., Mizuno K., 'Effects of thermal environment on sleep and circadian rhythm'. In: *Journal of Physiological Anthropology*, vol. 31:14.

×   Oliver, J., *Back care, an illustrated guide*, Butterworth-Heinemann, Oxford 1994.

×   Oliver, J. & A. Middleditch, *Functional anatomy of the spine*. Butterworth-Heinemann, Oxford 1991, pp. 295-316.

×   Oostendorp, R.A.B., 'De musculaire dysbalans bij de patiënt met lage rugklachten'. In: *Nederlands Tijdschrift voor Fysiotherapie* 90 (1980), pp. 82-89.

×   Oostendorp, R.A.B., 'Mobiliseren en/of immobiliseren van de lumbale wervelkolom en het belang van de propriosensoriek'. In: *De rug gesteund*. Leiden 1985, pp. 75-98.

×   Oosterhuis H.J.G.H., *Klinische neurologie – een beknopt leerboek*. Bohn, Scheltema& Holkema, Houten/Antwerpen, 1990.

×   Pande K.C., 'The role of bed rest in acute lower back pain'. In: *Journal of Indian Medical Association* (2004), 102 (4): 202-204, 208.

×   Panjabi, M.M., 'Kinematics of lumbar inter-vertebral foramen'. In: *Spine* 18 (1993).

×   Panjabi, M.M., V.K. Goel & K. Takata, 'Psysiologic strains in the lumbar spinal ligaments'. In: *Spine* 7 (1982), nr. 3, pp. 192-203.

×   Panjabi, M., A.A. White, W.O. Southwick et al., 'Effect of preload on load displacement curves of the lumbar spine'. In: *Orthopaedic Clinics of North America* (1977), nr. 8, pp. 181-192.

×   Parmeggiani P.L., 'REM sleep related increase in brain temperature: a physiologic problem'. In: *Archives Italiennes de Biologie* (2007), 145, pp. 13-21.

×   Pearson, D.J., 'Allergens and occlusive bedding'. In: *Lancet* 342 (1993), nr. 8869, pp. 494-495.

×   Penning, L. & T.J. Wilmink, 'Posture dependent bilateral compression of L4 or L5 nerve roots in facet hypertrophy: a dynamic CT-myelographic study'. In: *Spine* 12 (1987).

×   Persson L., Moritz U., 'Neck support pillows: a comparative study'. In: *Journal of Manipulative and Physiological Therapeutics* (1998), vol. 21, nr. 4, pp. 237-240.

×   Pheasant, S.T., *Ergonomics, work and health*. MacMillan Academy and Professional Ltd., London 1991.

×   Poortvliet, M.P., *Het beste bed voor de gezonde rug*. Eindexamenscriptie. Akademie voor Fysiotherapie Leffelaar, Amsterdam 1983.

×   Pope M.H., Hansson T.H., 'Vibration of the spine and lower back pain'. In: *Clinical Orthopedic Related Research* (1992), (279), pp. 49-59.

×   Pratap, H.J., 'Double beds and backache'. In: *Practitioner* 197 (1966), nr. 182. pp. 810-811.

×   Price P., Rees-Mathews S., Tebble NCamilleri J., 'The use of a new overlay mattress in patients with chronic pain impact on sleep and self-reported pain'. In: *Clinical Rehabilitation* (2003), 17 (5), pp. 488-492.

×   Purushothaman B., Singh A., Lingutla K., Bhatia C., Pollock R., Krishna M., 'Prevalence of insomnia in patients with chronic back pain'. In: *Journal of Orthopedic Surgery* (2013), 21(1), p. 68-70.

×   Quintet, R.J. & N.M. Hadler, 'Diagnosis and treatment of backache'. In: *Seminars in Arthritis and Rheumatism* (1979), nr. 8, pp. 261 -287.

×   Raebel, C., 'We hebben maar één rug en daar moeten we 't mee doen!' *Het ruggeboekje van Ubica*, 5e druk. Ubica Matrassen B.V., Utrecht 1988.

×   Ray J., 'Spine configuration associed with various sleep surfaces'. In: *IEEE Engineering in Medicine and Biology Magazine*, 10(2), pp. 33-36.

×   Raymann R.J.E.M., Swaab D.F., Van Someren E.J.W., 'Skin temperature and sleep-onset latency: changes with age and insomnia'. In: *Physiological Behav* (2007), 90, pp. 257-266.

×   Raymann R.J.E.M., Swaab D.F., Van Someren E.J.W., 'Skin deep: cutaneous temperature determines sleep depth'. In: *Brain* (2008) 131, pp. 500-513.

×   Raymann R.J.E.M., Van Someren E.J.W. 'Time-on-task impairment of psychomotor vigilance is affected by mild skin warming and changes with aging and insomnia'. In: *Sleep* (2007), 30, pp. 96-103.

×   Raymann R.J.E.M., Van Someren E.J.W., 'Diminished capability to recognize the optimal temperature for sleep initiation may contribute to poor sleep in elderly people'. In: *Sleep* (2008), 31, pp. 1301-1309.

×   Raymann RJ, Swaab DF., Van Someren EJ., 'Cutaneous warming promotes sleep onset'. In: *American Journal of Physiology* (2005) vol. 288 (6), pp. 1589-R1597.

×   Rebus, I., *De sterke rug: verzorging en herstel*. s.l. 1989.

×   Reichert, F.L., 'Compression of the brachial plexus: the scalene anticus syndrome'. In: *JAMA* (1942), nr. 118, pp. 294-295.

×   Rens, T.J.G. van, 'Lage rugklachten en lumbosacrale instabiliteit'. In: *Nederlands Tijdschrift voor Fysiotherapie* 90 (1980), nr. 3, pp. 74-81.

×   Reuber, M., 'Bulging of lumbar inter-vertebral discs'. In: *Journal of Biomechanical Engineering* (1982), nr. 104, pp. 187-192.

×   Ridder, A.J. de, 'De neurofysiologie van de pijn'. In: *Nederlands Tijdschrift voor Fysiotherapie* 95 (1985), nr. 6, pp. 141-143.

×   Rissanen, P.M., 'The surgical anatomy and pathology of the supraspinous and interspinous ligaments of the lumbar spine with special reference to ligament ruptures'. In: *Acta Orthopaedica Scandinavica* (1960), Suppl., p. 46.

×   Roeck, J. de & R. Matthys 'Het klinisch slaaponderzoek: Deel 1', *Tijdschrift voor Geneeskunde* 37 (1981), nr. 19, pp. 1145-1155.

×   Rombaut W., *Rug-en nekklachten klein krijgen*. Globe, 2000, Roeselare.

×   Romeijn N., Raymann R.J.E.M., Most E., et al., 'Sleep, vigilance, and thermosensitivity'. In: *Pflugers Arch.* (2012), vol. 463 (1), pp. 169-176.

×   Rompe, G., 'Orthopädie des Bettes'. In: *Österrreichische Krankenpflegezeitschrift* 36 (1983), nr. 4, pp. 117-119.

×   Ropponen A., Silventoinen K., Hublin C. et al., 'Sleep patterns as predictors for disability pension duet of lower back diagnoses: a 23-year longitudinal study of Finnish twins'. In: *Sleep* (2013), vol. 36, nr. 6, pp. 891-897.

×   Rosekind, M., Phillips, R., Rappaport J., et al., 'Effects of water bed surface on sleep'. In: *Sleep* (1976), res.5, 132.

×   Rozenberg S., Delval C. et al., 'Bed rest or normal activity for patients with acute lower back pain'. In: *Spine* (2000), vol. 27, nr. 14, pp. 1487-1493.

×   Rozenberg S., Allaert FA. et al., 'Compliance among general practitioners in France with recommendations not to prescribe bed rest for acute lower back pain'. In: *Joint Bone Spine* (2004), 71 (1), pp. 56-59.

×   Rubin, D., 'The no or the yes and the how of sex for patients with neck, back and radicular pain syndromes'. In: *Calif. Med.* (1970), 113, 6, pp. 12-15.

×   Salo et al. 'Effect of neck strength training on health-related quality of life in females with chronic neck pain: a randomized controlled 1-year follow-up study'. In: *Health and quality of life outcomes* (2010), 8 (48) pp. 1-7.

×   Salvetti M., et al., Prevalencia y factores asociados con la fatiga en patients con dolor lumbar cronico'. In: *Revista Latino-Americano de Enfermagem* (2013) vol. 21.

×   Sandover, J., 'Dynamic loading as a possible source of low-back pain'. In: *Spine* 8 (1983), nr. 6, pp. 652-658.

×   Saunders, H.D., 'Lumbale tractie'. In: G.P. Grieve (ed.), *Moderne manuele therapie van de wervelkolom* (deel 2), De Tijdstroom, Lochem 1989, pp. 832-839.

×   Scharf M.B., Stover R., McDannold M., Kaye H., Berkowitz D.V., 'Comparative effects of sleep on a standard mattress to an experimental foam surface on sleep architecture and CAP rates'. In: *Sleep* (1997), (20), pp. 1197-1200.

×   Schut, G.L., 'Preventie van decubitus'. In: *Tijdschrift voor Ziekenverpleging* 37 (1984), nr. 6, pp. 162-175.

×   Schneider, N.N. & D. Helmert, 'Schlafstörungen – ein Problem unserer Zeit'. In: *Schweizerische Aerzte Zeitung* (1985), nr. 66, pp. 1102-1108.

×   Schonstrom, N.S.R., 'The pathomorfology of spinal stenosis as seen on CT-scans of the lumbar spine'. In: *Spine* 10 (1985), nr. 9, pp. 806-811.

×   Schreuder, K.E, *The effect of cervical positioning on benign snoring by means of a custom-fitted pillow*, The Netherlands.

×   Seysener, M., 'Decubitus: oorzaken, preventie en behandeling'. In: *MGZ* 15 (1987), nr. 12, pp. 24-27.

×   Shan X., Ning X., et al., 'Lower back pain development response to sustained trunk axial twisting'. In: *European Spine Journal* (2013), 22, pp. 1972-1978.

×   Shanmugan B., Roux F., Stonestreet C. et al., 'Lower back pain and sleep: mattresses, sleep quality and daytime symptoms'. In: *Sleep Diagnosis and Therapy* (2007), vol. 2, nr. 5, pp. 36-40.

×   Shapiro, C.M., A.T. Moore & D. Mitchell, 'How well does man thermoregulate during sleep?'. In: *Experientia* 30 (1974), nr. 11, pp. 1279-1281.

×   Siebke, H.J., *Möbel für den Schlafbereich*. Abschlußarbeit. Fachhochschule Lippe, Lippe 1979.

×   Sjögren, K. & A.R. Fugl-Meyer, 'Chronic back pain and sexuality'. In: *International Rehabilitation Medicine* 3 (1981), nr. 1, pp. 19-25.

×   Smits, M.G., 'Hoe kan een acuut optredende ischialgie worden verklaard?' *Vademecum permanente bijscholing huisartsen* 8, 1990, 11p.

×   Smot, P., E. Schrier & H.W.J. Wilms, 'Immobilisatie: gevolgen voor spier- en botweefsel'. In: *Nederlands Tijdschrift voor Fysiotherapie* 98 (1988), nr. 1, pp. 11-17.

×   Smythe, H., 'Fibrositis and soft tissue pain syndromes'. In: I.V.J. Malcolm (ed.), *The lumbar spine and back pain*, 3rd edition, Churchill Livingstone, New York 1987, pp. 402-418.

×   Snijders, G.J., 'Liggen'. In: *Biomechanica van het skeletsysteem, grondslagen en toepassingen*. De Tijdstroom, Lochem/Gent, pp. 367-372.

×   Sofres (Frans instituut voor opiniepeilingen). 'Les francais et la literie'. In: *Annales de Kinésithérapie* 15 (1988), nr. 3, pp. 113-118.

× Staes F., Brumagne S., *Kinesitherapeutisch onderzoek van onderste extremiteiten en lumbale wervelkolom*. Acco, Leuven/Den Haag, 2011.

× Stankovic, R. & O. Johnell, 'Conservative treatment of acute low-back pain: a prospective randomized trial. McKenzie method of treatment versus patient education in "mini back school"'. In: *Spine* 15 (1990), nr. 2, pp. 120-123.

× Stappaerts, K. & D. Everaert, *Pas op!... je rug!: preventie van rugklachten*, ilo, Leuven 1992.

× Steeno, O.P. & A. Pangkahila, 'Occupational influences on male fertility and sexuality'. In: *Andrologia* 16 (1984), nr. 2, pp. 93-98.

× Stevens, J., 'Lower back pain'. In: *Medical Clinics of North America* (1968), nr. 52, pp. 55-71.

× Stijns, H.J., *Klinisch onderzoek van het bewegingsstelsel*. Acco, Leuven 1986.

× Struyf-Denys, G., *Précautions, prévention et réadaptation pour les souffrants de la colonne vertébrale*. Prodim, Bruxelles 1978 s.p.

× Sung EJ., Tochihara Y., 'Effects of Bathing and Hot Footbath on Sleep in Winter'. In: *Journal of Physiological Anthropology and Applied Human Science* (1999), pp. 21-27.

× Svenonius, E., A.L. Hojerback & G. Landquist (eds.), 'A mattress cover relieves mite allergy'. In: *Lakartidningen* 90 (1993), nr. 4, pp. 264-265.

× Swart, M.E., *Anti-decubitus ligondersteuning*. Afstudeerverslag tussenafdeling Industrieel Ontwerpen, tu Delft, maart 1983.

× Swezey, R.L. & P.J. Clement, 'Conservative treatment of back pain'. In: I.V.J. Malcolm (ed.), *The lumbar spine and back pain* , 3rd edition, Churchill Livingstone, New York 1987, pp. 300-314.

× Tamura, T., T. Togawa & M. Murata, 'A bed temperature monitoring system for assessing body movements during sleep'. In: *Clinical Physics & Physiological Measurement* 9 (1988), nr. 2, pp. 139-145.

× Tanner, J. & G.T. Haneveld, *Rugklachten: voorkomen en genezen*. Zomer & Keuning, Ede/ Antwerpen 1988.

× Ten Holte-de Vries N., M.G. Smits & A.H.M. Wolswijk, 'Een klinische bedrustkuur bij hernia-patiënten'. In: *Tijdschrift voor Ziekenverpleging* (1991), nr. 17, pp. 606-609.

× Testaankoop, Verbruikersunie. Dossier met algemeen deel technisch rapport aan P. Mannekens, Brussel. Privé-verzameling P. Coninck, getypt, Brussel 1991.

× Testaankoop, *Veermatrassen* (2013), nr. 572 p.24-27.

× Tetley M., 'Instinctive sleeping and resting postures: an anthropological and zoological approach to treatment of lower back and joint pain'. In: *British Medical Journal* (2000), 321, pp. 1616-1618.

× Tollison, C.D. & M.L. Kniegel, *Interdisciplinary rehabilitation of lower back pain*. Williams & Wilkins, Baltimore 1989.

× Torrance, C., 'Pressure sores pathogenesis'. In: *Nursing Times* (1981), nr. 3, p. 3.

× Tortora, G.J. & N.P. Anagnestakes, *Principles of anatomy and physiology*, 5th edition, Harper & Row, New York 1987.

× Toshihiko, M., D. Osborne, D.W. Swanson & J.M. Halling, 'Chronic pain patients and spouses: marital and sexual adjustment'. In: *Mayo Clinic Proceedings* (1981), nr. 56, pp. 307-310.

× Touchon, 'Réaction du spécialiste du sommeil'. In: *Ann, Kinésither* 15 (1988) nr. 3, pp. 119-120.

× Tovey, E. & G. Marks (eds.), 'Allergens and occlusive bedding covers'. In: *Lancet* 342 (1993), nr. 8863, pp. 126-127.

×   Tracey, J.B., 'The wheat bed and cushions in general practice'. In: *Practitioner* 204 (1970), nr. 224, pp. 845-846.

×   Travell, J.G. & D.G. Simons, *Myofascial pain and dysfunction: the trigger point manual* (volume 2), Williams & Wilkins, Baltimore 1992.

×   Twomey, L.T. & J.R. Taylor, *Physical therapy of the lower back*, 2nd edition, Churchill Livingstone, New York 1994.

×   Twomey, L.T. & J.R. Taylor, 'Sagittal movements of the human vertebral column: a quantitive study of the role of the posterior vertebral elements'. In: *Archives of Physical Medicine & Rehabilitation* 64 (1983), pp. 322-323.

×   Unger, H., 'Zur Lagerungsbehandlung von Wirbelsäulenerkrankungen'. In: *Münchener Medizinische Wochenschrift* 112 (1970), nr. 50, pp. 2292-2293.

×   Vallen, V., 'Potential for bed sores due to high pressures: influence of body sites, body position, and mattress design'. In: *BJCP* 47 (1993), pp. 195-197.

×   Valtonen, E.J., 'Rücken und bett'. In: *Lakartidningen* 76 (1979), nr. 38, pp. 3177-3179.

×   Vandegriend B., Hill D., Raso J., Durdle N., Zhang Z., 'Application of computer graphics for assessment of spinal deformities'. In: *Medical and Biological Engineering Computing* (1995), 33, pp. 163-166.

×   Vandenboorn, H.J.M., 'Voorlichting over lig-/slaaphoudingen en bedden: voldoende onderbouwd?'. In: *Tijdschrift voor Ergonomie* (1993), pp. 1-6.

×   Van de Water A.T., Eadie J., Hurley D.A., 'Investigation of sleep disturbance in chronic lower back pain: an age-and gender-matched case-control study over a 7-night period'. In: *Manual Therapy* (2011), 16 (6), pp. 550-556.

×   Vanharanta, H., 'The relationship of pain provocation to lumbar disc deterioration.' In: *Spine* 12 (1987), nr. 3, pp. 295-298.

×   Van Nugteren K., Winkel D., *Onderzoek en behandeling van de nek*. Bohn Stafleu van Loghum, Houten, 2012.

×   Van Someren E.J.W., 'Sleep propensity is modulated by circadian and behavior-induced changes in cutaneous temperature'. In: *Journal Therm. Biol.* (2004), 29, pp. 437-444.

×   Van Someren E.J.W., 'Mechanics and functions of coupling between sleep and temperature rhythms'. In: *Prog. Brain Res.* (2006), 153, pp. 309-324.

×   Van Tulder M.W., Koes B.W., Assendelft W.J.J., Bouter L.M., Daams, Van der Laan J.R., 'Acute lage rugpijn: actief blijven, NSAID's en spierverslappers effectief, bedrust en specifieke oefeningen niet effectief; resultaten van systematische reviews'. In: *Nederlands Tijdschrift voor Geneeskunde* (2000), 144, (31), pp. 1489-1494.

×   Verbraecken J., Bergen T., *S.O.S. Slaap*, Houtekiet, Antwerpen, 2014.

×   Verbraecken J., Buyse B., Hamburger H., Van Kasteel V., Van Steenwijk R., *Leerboek Slaap en slaapstoornissen*. Acco, Leuven/ Den Haag, 2013.

×   Verhaert V., Haex B., De Wilde T., Berckmans D., Verbraecken J., de Valck E., Vander Sloten J., 'Ergonomics in bed design: the effect of spinal alignment on sleep parameters'. In: *Ergonomics* (2011), vol. 54, nr. 2, pp. 169-178.

×   Verhaert V., De Bruyne G., De Wilde T. et al. 'Bed temperature and humidity during sleep in mild thermal conditions'. In: *Sleep* (2011), vol. 34, A109, abstract supplement nr. 0310.

×   Verwimp, A., *Bedcomfort voor ruglijders: evaluatie van vier verschillende matrasdragers*. Licentiaats-verhandeling motorische revalidatie en kinesitherapie. ku Leuven, Leuven 1989.

×   Visser, P. & W.F. Hofman, 'Slapen en dromen: theorie en klinische praktijk'. In: *De Nederlandse bibliotheek der geneeskunde*, deel 181, jaargang 21. Samsom Stafleu, Alphen aan den Rijn/Brussel 1986.

×   Vleeming A., Albert H.B., Ostgaard H.C., Sturesson B., Stuge B., 'European guidelines for the diagnosis and treatment of pelvic girdle pain'. In: *European Spine Journal*, DOI 10.1007/s00586-008-0602-4.

×   Voermans, F, 'Enige verkenningen naar het gebruik van "The Pillow"'. In: *Belgisch Tijdschrift voor Fysische Therapie* (1983), nr. 3, pp. 109-111.

×   Voldere, J. de, Document aan P. Mannekens over het bed. Leeuwarden 7/7/1993, (18 p.). Privé-verzameling dr. J. de Voldere, Heerenveen.

×   Voldere, J. de, *Leven zonder rugklachten: oorzaken, tips behandeling*. Van Gorcum, Assen 1978.

×   Vojta P.J., Randels S.P. et al. 'Effects of physical interventions on house dust mite allergen levels in carpet, bed, and upholstery dust in low-income, urban homes'. In: *Environmental Health Perspectives* (2001), vol. 109, nr. 8, pp. 815-819.

×   Vries, J. de, *De natuurlijke aanpak van nek- en rugklachten*, Kosmos, Utrecht 1992.

×   Waddell G., Feder G., Lewis M., 'Systematic reviews of bed rest and advice to stay active for acute lower back pain'. In: *British Journal of General Practice* (1997), 47, pp. 647-652.

×   White, A. & R. Anderson, 'Conservative care of lower back pain'. In: N.C. Selby, *Basic back school concept*, s.l., (s.a.), pp. 39-44.

×   White, A.A. & M.M. Panjabi, *Clinical biomechanics of the spine*. J.B. Lippincott Company, Philadelphia 1978.

×   Wierinckx, A., *Ergonomie en hygiëne van het wonen*, s.l., s.a., pp. 105-122.

×   Wijmen, P.M. van, 'Lumbale pijnsyndromen'. In: G.P. Grieve (red.), *Moderne manuele therapie van de wervelkolom* (deel 1), De Tijdstroom, Lochem 1988, pp. 476-494.

×   Wilke H.J., Neef P., Caimi M., Hoogland T., Claes L.E., 'New in vivo measurements of pressures in the inter-vertebral disc in daily life'. In: *Spine* (1999), vol.24 (8), pp. 755-762.

×   Wilke H.J., *Ergomechanics 2, Interdisciplinary Conference on Spinal Column Research*, Shaker, Aachen, 2010.

×   Wilkinson M.J., 'Does 48 hours' bed rest influence the outcome of acute lower back pain?' In: *British Journal of General Practice* (1995), 45, pp. 481-484.

×   Williams, P.C., *The lumbosacral spine: emphasizing conservative management*, McGraw-Hill, New York 1965.

×   Williams, R.L. & I. Karakan (eds.), 'The electroencephalogram sleep patterns of middle-aged males'. In: *Journal of Nervous & Mental Disease*, vol. 154 (1972), nr. 1, pp. 22-30.

×   Winkel, D., *Informatie voor mensen met rugklachten*, Bohn Stafleu Van Loghum, Houten 1991.

×   Winkel, D., G. Aufdemkampe & O.H. Meijer, *Orthopedische geneeskunde en manuele therapie: diagnostiek extremiteiten* (deel 2), Bohn Stafleu Van Loghum, Houten 1992.

×   Wisconsin Alumni Research Foundation, 'Cotton or latex mattresses? A bacteriological evaluation of latex foam rubber'. In: *Canadian Hospital* (1967), pp. 70-74.

×   Wittig, R.M. & F.J. Zorick (eds.), 'Distributed sleep in patients complaining of chronic pain'. In: *Journal of Nervous & Mental Disease* 170 (1982), nr. 429.

×   Wolf, A.N. de, *Achter de rug?: alles over rugklachten*, Bohn Scheltema & Holkema, Utrecht, 1989.

×   Wolfe, F, 'Fibrositis, fibromyalgia, and musculoskeletal disease: the current status of the fibrositis syndrome'. In: *Archives of Physical Medicine & Rehabilitation*, 69 (1988), pp. 527-531.

×   Wurff, P. van der, 'Preventie en behandeling van decubitus'. In: *Tijdschrift voor Ziekenverpleging* 43 (1989), nr. 13, pp. 425-428.

×   Xhardez, Y. & V. Cloquet, *Verrouillage et protection de la colonne dorso-lombaire: précis pratiques de rééducation*. Frison-Roche, Paris 1990.

×   Zimmerman, W.B., 'Sleep mentation and auditory awakening threshold'. In: *Psychophysiology* (1970), nr. 6, pp. 540-549.

×   Zito, M., Driver D., Parker C., 'Lasting effects of one bout of two 15-seconds passive stretches on ankle dorsiflexion range of motion'. In: *Journal of Orthopedic&Sports Physical Therapy*, (1997), vol. 26 (4), pp. 114-221.

Useful websites

www.cost.eu
Website of the European Corporation in Science and Technology COST ACTION B13 which issues guidelines regarding the treatment of lower back pain. The website is for professionals involved in the multidisciplinary treatment of back patients. The links are interesting, with references to scientific journals and articles. When filling in 'back pain' in the search bar, you will get some interesting information.

www.bettersleep.org
The official website of the BSC (Better Sleep Council), the non-profit organisation founded in 1979 by the American mattress industry. This is an informative website for the general public with more explanation about the importance of good sleep and a good night's rest for your health. The section headed 'Better Sleep' is nice to read sometime.

www.chiropractic-uk.co.uk
Website of the British Association of Chiropractors. Packed with useful information for back patients. Going to the home page and clicking on 'for everyone', you can look at the section: Mind your posture/ Buying a bed/ Sleeping.

www.nomite.de

Informative website of the German Federation of Down and Feathers for patients with house dust allergy. Many useful tips on purchase and maintenance of bed linen. Also suitable for professionals, in view of the link to scientific articles about house dust mites and bed linen. Nomite is a quality mark.

www.sleepcouncil.org.uk

Website of the British mattress federation, the National Bed Federation of the UK. Go to the homepage and click on 'bed advice'. Look after your back – choose the right bed. At the right side of this page you can find useful links, many sleep tips and informative videos.

www.backcare.org.uk

This website was established by Staley Grundly in 1968, after his own back injury, caused by a sailing accident mainly due to the lack of information and support for back pain sufferers during this time.

When opening the website, go to Library and fill out the keyword 'bed'. You will see a PDF with relevant information about beds and mattresses.

www.sleepdex.org/hygiene.htm

Website of Dan Crean. No-nonsense approach with a lot of content about everything on the theme of sleep. The website is also very useful for professionals with several links to scientific articles.

www.sleepfoundation.org

Website of the American Sleep Foundation. Very professional content and useful for anyone who wants to know more about 'sleep'. Also relevant links to scientific articles for professionals.

www.allergyuk.org

Allergy UK is the leading national charity dedicated to supporting the estimated 21 million allergy sufferers in the UK. They provide a dedicated 'getting-help/allergy-uk-helpline' helpline, support network and online 'http://forum.allergyuk.org/' forum for those with allergy.

Interesting to read is the information about house dust mites and controlling house dust mite allergens at home.

www.spine-health.com

Magnificent website about everything you need to know about your back! Probably the best in the world. A great deal of information, and very instructive with several videos. Among other things, the website gives you an overview of types of back pain, treatments, wellness, pain forums, and the like. The videos are very useful to have a look at, because some are accompagnied by exercises. Discuss the exercises first with your occupational therapist/physical therapist. There is also a link provided for professionals.

www.edfa.eu

The European Down and Feather Association, EDFA is established on 11.11.1990 by nine companies from eight different countries with headquaters in Frankfurt.

When opening the website, go to Consumer Information. Here you can find information about Sleeping climate/ Buying tips/ Care Tips.

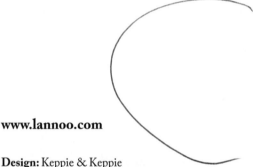

www.lannoo.com

Design: Keppie & Keppie
Binnenwerk: Wim De Dobbeleer
Cover photo: © Image Source/Corbis
Illustrations inside: © Frank Geisler, Marc Jacops
Translation: Madeline Cohen

© Lannoo Publishers, Tielt, 2016 and Pascal Mannekens
D/2016/45/529 − NUR 860
ISBN 978 94 014 3937 4

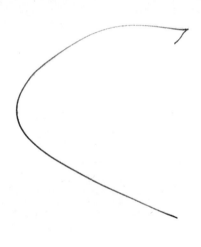